Fitness by Penis

www.fitnessbypenis.com

Peter Pandore

Fitness by Penis

Panarex Productions
Peter Pandore

Third Edition
2007

ISBN
978-1-4116-9912-0
0-9780897-0-7

BE BOTH PROUD OF YOUR BODY AND SIZE!

**Innovative, easy and healthy exercises
to build your muscles while enlarging your penis.**

**It is Natural
It is Healthy
It is Fun**

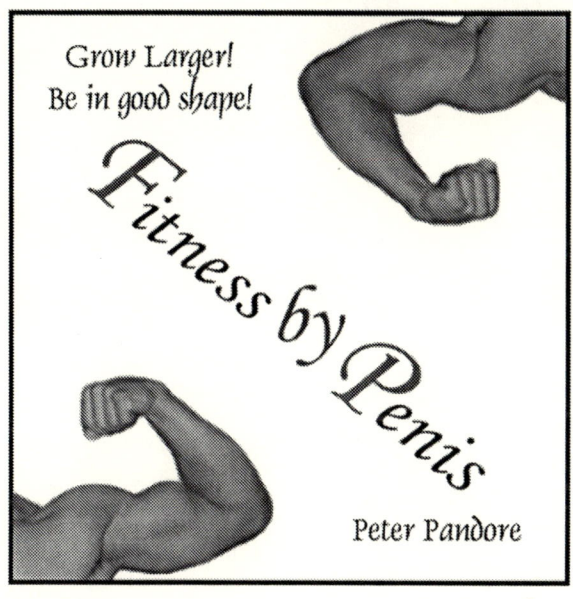

Grow Larger!
Be in good shape!

Fitness by Penis

Peter Pandore

TABLE OF CONTENTS

EXERCISES

Section 1

1- Warm-up Fist Exercise
2- Warm-up Shoulder Pull
3- Up and Down
4- Vertical Circular Movement
5- Horizontal Circular Movement
6- Shoulder Twist
7- Waist Twist
8- Multiple Pull

9- In and Out
10- Under Leg
11- Over Leg
12- Both Hands Back Pull
13- One Hand Back Pull
14- Bend Stretch – A
15- Bend Stretch – B
16- Foot Workout
17- Legs Workout
18- Bend Pull
19- Side Stretch – A
20- Side Stretch – B
21- Twist Stretch
22- Gear Pull
23- Rolling Exercise
24- Spinning Exercise
25- Fold Exercise
26- Fold Fist Exercise
27- Cross Stretch
28- Crank Exercise

Section 2

29- Sit-up Stretch
30- Leg Pull
31- Leg Side Pull
32- Lower Back Stretch
33- Legs up Pull

Section 3

34- Jelq Technique (Milking)
35- Inflation Exercise
36- Stroke Exercise
37- Downward Milking
38- Under Leg Milking
39- Behind Milking
40- Bend Milking

DISCLAIMER

The exercises in this manual are designed based on the highest safety and comfort consideration for the user, and they have been practiced by the author for many years. Depending on your body's strength, you are in charge of choosing which of these exercises are safe and suitable for your body. Some people can handle the roughest exercises when enlarging their penis and developing their muscles while some might be challenged even with the simplest one. Fitness by Penis, like any other body workout, has to be practiced according to safety procedures. Any misuse of these practices and escaping safety procedures written in the introduction of this manual and in the exercises can lead to harming your genital and muscles.

You should be aware that these exercises might not be suitable for those with illnesses that may alter blood circulation, oxygenation, and regeneration of tissues. Examples of these diseases are advanced diabetes, respiratory instability, cirrhosis, genitourinary disorders and hypertension. Before engaging in any of the exercises or dietary procedures mentioned in this manual consult with your doctor and/or urologist to make sure that using the contents of this manual is suitable for your body.

By reading this legal notice and practicing the exercises contained in this manual you declare that the author of these exercises and fitnessbypenis.com or their parent company(s) and any individual(s) affiliated with the production company are not responsible for ANY damage and injury to your genitals, body and mental health that may occur directly or indirectly by use or misuse of the contents or exercises contained within, and you take full responsibility for any possible injury and health problem(s).

INTRODUCTION

In this manual, you will learn to use your penis as the most effective tool to shape your body and also to add extra thickness and length to your penis.

FITNESS BY PENIS is the right method that you were always looking for. It is designed to help you achieve a healthy and strong body along with even a healthier and stronger sexual drive and penis.

Here is the good news to inspire and excite you to go for your dreams in achieving a Super Large Penis and Athletic Muscles. Both your muscles and penis share the same function and purpose, which is GROWING and ENLARGING. Therefore, your muscles and penis, due to their nature, would demand exercises that can help them grow thicker, longer and stronger. In addition, since your penis becomes erect by absorbing blood in its spongy chambers, it can be enlarged by increasing the capacity of its spongy tissues. In order to achieve a larger penis and stronger muscles you do not need to practice all the exercises. From the forty given exercises choose the best ones that suit your body, and by practicing the exercises in this manual for ten to fifteen minutes a day you will witness the growth of your muscles and penis in a couple of weeks. It is important to decide which exercises are the ones you can perform on a daily basis and you can stick to them. For example, you might find out that the exercises that you can do regularly are those which can be done while taking your daily shower. In addition to all the exercises there are many tips on nutrition, mental health, penis anatomy, preparation, penile abuse, sex drive and erection that can help you achieve your goal and fulfill your dream more efficiently and quickly.

It is a fact that without daily activity and exercises we are very likely to have high cholesterol, heart disease, blockage of the arteries, prostate and colon cancer and many other diseases that can shorten our life. If you are also concerned about the health, strength and the size of your penis, **FITNESS BY PENIS** is the best healthy and safe method to help you achieve your goal and to gain both an athletic body and a larger penis at the same time.

HOW TO OPTIMIZE
PENIS AND MUSCLE ENLARGEMENT

1- Your penis and muscles are parts of your body that share the same physical purpose and function. They are both optimized to achieve more strength and mass and eventually become larger.

2- With your daily ten to fifteen minutes exercise routine, five days a week, you can mostly see a noticeable gain in both your penis and body muscles within two weeks.

3- Your penis consists of three spongy chambers, which serve to absorb blood in order to become erect, and the key to have a larger penis is to expand these spongy tissues by given exercises in this manual.

4- Apply concentration, mental visualization and deep breathing to your exercises in order to reduce the risk of injury and to achieve a better result.

5- Be gentle with your penis and do the exercises moderately. Gentle daily exercise is a guaranteed procedure for a long lasting healthy workout.

6- Do not force your penis to have extra tolerance under pressure and tension. Excess of force over your penis can damage its tissues and bodies, and results in longer period of time for achieving a larger penis.

7- After each exercise or a set of exercises, take a break to heal and rejuvenate your muscles and tissues. Your penis grows through the process of cells splitting. This process necessitates enough time, nutrition and right physical and mental conditions.

8- If you feel any discomfort or notice any odd deformations, discolorations, spots and injuries on your penis stop exercising until the penis is completely back to its normal state.

9- If you do not feel safe in any exercise do not continue it and pick another one that suits you.

10- Whenever you are sick or you feel weak do the exercises more moderately and in shorter time to prevent exhaustion in your muscles and genitals.

HOW TO PREPARE BEFORE EACH EXERCISE

1- Keep your pubic hair short to facilitate the handling of your penis and also to help with sanitation.

2- It is always a good idea to stimulate yourself before daily exercises so that your testosterone level and your mental concentration on your genital increases, and you are ready for muscle development.

3- Before engaging in any exercise always warm up with a hot water-soaked towel or warm water. Then start with light and moderate exercises to avoid injuries to your penis and muscles.

4- Remember not to exercise right after ejaculation since your blood testosterone levels drop and all your connective tissues begin to tighten.

5- For lubrication, avoid any oil-based, chemical and artificial-based lubricant such as petroleum jelly, Vaseline, baby oil, hand lotion or any other cleaning agent. Use only natural lubricants that are suitable for your body.

ESSENTIAL FACTORS

1- Eat healthy, low fat, high-fiber food and include fruits and vegetables in your daily diet. Eat organic food as much as possible. Avoid animal fat, junk foods, fast foods, fried foods, processed foods, caned fruits and foods, artificial colors and flavors, pops, artificial sweeteners, excess of sugar, salt and condiments, and above all avoid smoking and drink alcohol in moderation.

2- You need certain vitamins and minerals to reform, rebuild and expand your penis and muscles in both length and volume. If necessary take a moderate supplement of minerals, amino acids and vitamins.

3- Drink daily at least eight cups of filtered water (preferably ozone-treated) and pure natural fruit juices in total.

4- Perform on a regular basis the daily given exercises. Daily exercises enhance your stamina, reduce your blood vessels' clogs (also called atherosclerosis), decrease body's total cholesterol and fat, improve blood circulation and make all your muscles stronger and healthier. They also help you maintain a good erection and provide you with more strength for a longer lasting sexual activity.

5- Mental relaxation and peace of mind are among the most important factors to increase the ability of your body in developing and maintaining sexual organs and hormones. Avoid stress as much as you can and occupy yourself with activities that bring meaning to your life and make you feel good about yourself and your surrounding environment.

SYMPTOMS OF PENILE ABUSE

Blisters:
Caused by severe pressure on the penis for a long period of time.

Red Sores:
As a result of too much stretch.

Blue Spots:
A consequence of bleeding directly into the skin which results in a few or many tiny bruises. They are not permanent and will slowly disappear in a few days.

Nerve Inflammation:
Occurs when too much weight is placed on the penis for a long period of time; this distorts the nerves and causes them to swell. It also reduces the ability to achieve an erection.

Fuzzy Skin:
External tissue abuse caused by too much tension on penis, and it is partially dead tissue covering the penis.

"If you notice any symptoms stop the exercise immediately and discontinue until the penis is healed and the symptoms are gone. If after several days symptoms still persist contact your doctor immediately."

THE ANATOMY OF PENIS

Anatomically male genitalia consist of a penis, two testicles, two sets of genital ducts and associated glands. The penis consists of three spongy chambers, which serve to absorb blood in order to become erected and expanded.

ANATOMY DEFINITIONS

Cavernous Urethra:
The canal through which urine passes from the bladder, and sperm from the testicles.

Corpus Cavernosum:
Two spongy chambers, which serve to absorb blood in order to become erect.

Corpus Spongiosum:
Spongy chamber, which serve to absorb blood in order to become erect.

Cowper's Glands:
The source of Mucoid Fluid (pre-sperm fluid)

Ejaculation Fluid:
A fluid consisting of 5% Sperm, 40% fluid from Prostate and 45% from Seminal Vesicles.

Ejaculatory Ducts:
A place through which the sperm and Seminal Vesicle fluid flow into the Urethra during ejaculation.

Epididymis:
A place in which sperms remain for about three weeks until they reach maturity.

Seminal Vesicles:
Generate fluid that acts as a nutrient in keeping the sperm healthy.

Testicles:
Two glands, which produce male hormones and sperm (seed).

Vas Deferens:
Tubes attached to the Epididymis carrying sperm to be stored in Ampulae.

Uretra
Bladder
Seminal Vesicles
Openings of Ejaculatory Duct
Cowper's Gland
Corpus Cavenosum
Cavernous Urethra
Epididymis
Testicle
Corpus Songiosum
Glans Penis

Front

Prostate
Pubic Bone
Corpus Cavenosum
Vas Deferens
Bladder
Seminal Vesicles
Ejaculatory Duct
Openings of E. Duct
Corpus Songiosum
Rectum
Cavernous Urethra
Epididymis
Muscle
Testicle
Cowper's Gland

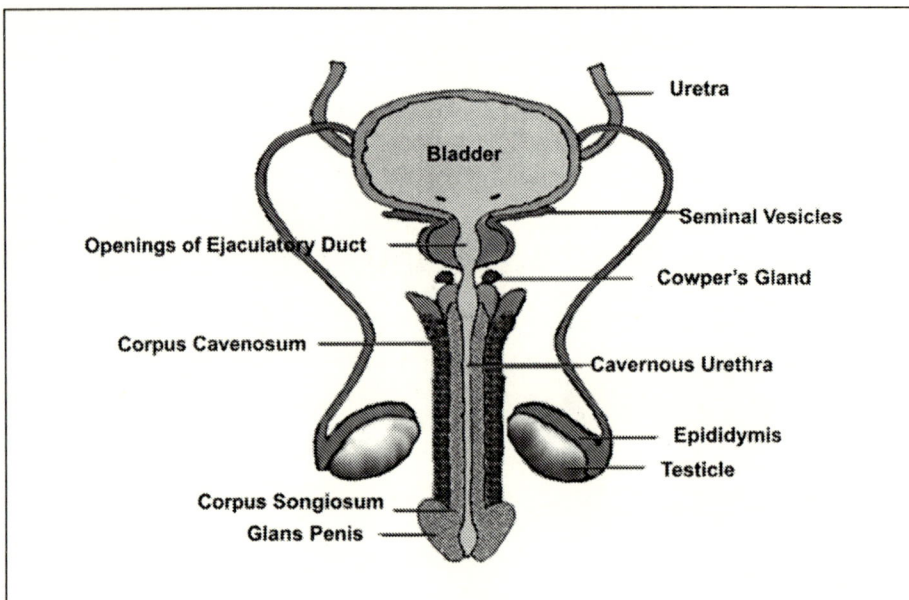

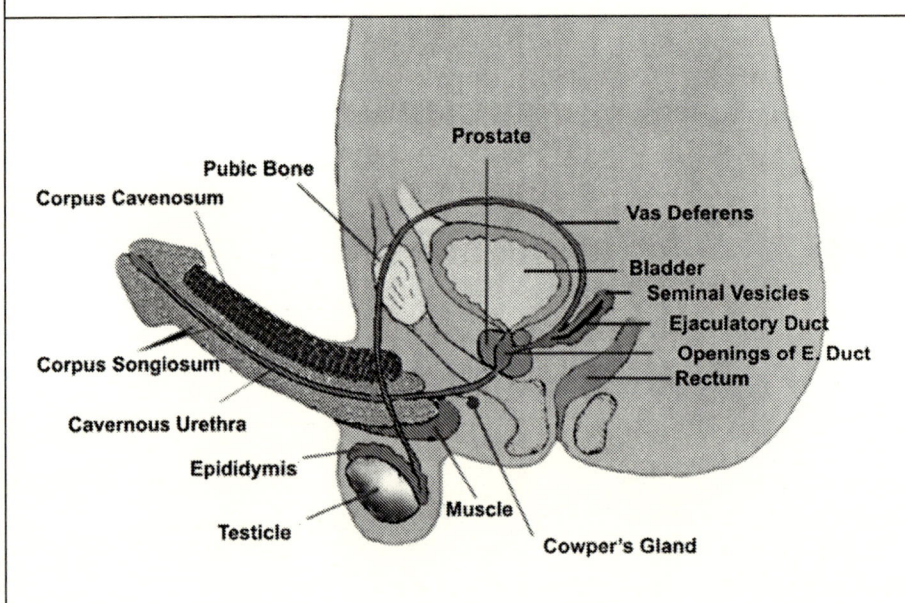

Side

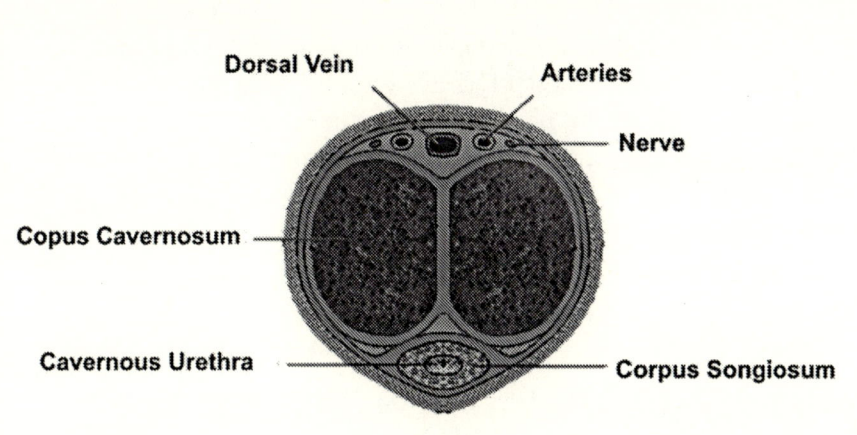

Dorsal Vein

Arteries

Nerve

Copus Cavernosum

Cavernous Urethra

Corpus Songiosum

Cross Section

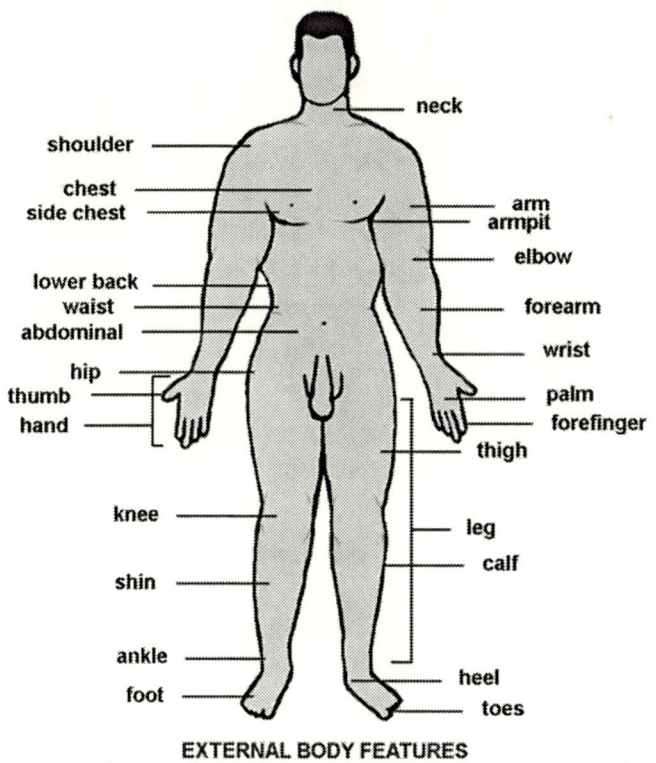

neck

shoulder

chest
side chest

arm
armpit

elbow

lower back
waist
abdominal

forearm

wrist

hip
thumb
hand

palm
forefinger

thigh

knee

leg

calf

shin

ankle
foot

heel

toes

EXTERNAL BODY FEATURES

17

SEX DRIVE AND HEALTHY PROSTATE FACTORS

A healthy sexual performance depends on many factors in our life style and diet. Some of the factors are scientifically proven and some are based on folklore and personal experiences. Here are some of the common and important considerations in improving a man's sexual performance.

INCREASING SEXUAL DESIRE
(Factors and Conditions)

Relaxation, Exercise, Healthy nutrition, Happiness, Massage, Kissing, Dancing, Sensual clothing, Sex fantasy visualization, Watching porn, Dirty talking and Sexual fantasy.

Pheromone: (odorless chemicals produced by body to sexually stimulate the opposite sex): Human pheromones are concealed in small quantities in skin oils around the nipples, under the armpit and near the genital region. Some synthetic pheromones are found in perfumes, colognes, aftershaves, candles or even in flavored lingerie.

Essential Oils: Some of essential oils have seducing effect

Hormonal Supplements: (only with doctor's consultations) DHEA (DeHyDroEpiAndrosterone), Pregnenolone, Testosterone a.k.a., Androstenedione, Natural Progesterone, Tibolone, Human Growth Hormone.

DECREASING SEXUAL DESIRE
(Factors and Conditions)

Anxiety, Stress, Overwork, Depression, Fatigue, Illness, Poor diet, Heavy meals , Shortage of sleep, Obesity, Anaemia, Prescribed drugs, Hyperprolactinaemia, Low male hormone level (testosterone), Alcoholism, Drugs abuse, and any major 'generalized' disease, such as Diabetes.

EDIBLE APHRODISIACS
(Information on many sex drive enhancing foods, fruits and vegetables)
"based on folklore"

Aniseed:
The seedlike fruit of the anise; an annual, aromatic Mediterranean herb in the parsley family. An aphrodisiac since the Greeks and the Romans. Sucking on the seeds increases sexual desire. Sleep-inducing and expectorant.

Almond:
An ancient symbol of fertility. It contains folate, vitamin E, A, niacin, , potassium, phosphorus, calcium, sodium, magnesium, selenium, iron, zinc and manganese.

Apple:
Symbol of sexuality. It awakens passion in men. It is high in dietary fiber and vitamin A, C, E, folate (important during pregnancy), potassium, calcium, phosphorus, magnesium and selenium.

Arugula ("Rocket"seed):
From a Mediterranean plant. An aphrodisiac since the first century A.D. Also its leaves are used in salad and pasta. It was added to grated orchid bulbs and parsnips and also, it was combined with pistachios and pine nuts.

Asparagus:
A good source of vitamin A, C, niacin, folate, potassium, phosphorus, calcium, sodium, magnesium and fiber. It is more effective in boosting sexual desire if eating it for three days.

Avocado:
Rich in vitamin A, B1(thiamine), B2 (riboflavin), B6, C, niacin, folate, pantothenic acid, potassium, phosphorus, magnesium, calcium, sodium and iron. It is also high in folic acid, dietary fiber and glutamine "antioxidant". Also important during pregnancy and formation of the baby's neural tube.

Betel Palm:
The seed of a tropical Asian feather-leaved palm. Used in brahmanic tradition, and contains alkaloids that stimulates entire body.

Banana:
Necessary for sex hormone production. A milkshake with banana increases arousal. Rich in vitamin A, C, B6, E, folate, niacin, pantothenic acid, potassium, magnesium, phosphorus, calcium, selenium and iron.

Carrots:
A good source of vitamin A, C, B6, niacin, folate, pantothenic acid, potassium, sodium, calcium, phosphorus, magnesium and iron.

Cashews:
A good source of vitamin K, folate, potassium, phosphorus, manganese, calcium, Sodium, iron, zinc and selenium.

Caviar:
Rich in vitamin B6, B5, B2, B12, A,C, PP and phosphorus.

Celery:
A good source of vitamin K, C, B6, B1, A, B2, folate, potassium, dietary fiber, manganese, calcium, magnesium, phosphorus and iron. Boosts monkeys' multiple ejaculations for up to seven times a day!

Chilies:
Stimulating spice. Rich in vitamin A, C, E, fiber, potassium, iron and folic acid.

Coriander (Cilantro seed):
An aromatic annual Eurasian herb in the parsley family. An ancient aphrodisiac and appetite stimulant. Mentioned in the ancient book of the Arabian Nights.

Chocolate 'dark':
Its caffeine and theobromine stimulate romance and desire. Contains antioxidant; an cancer preventing enzymes.

Cucumber:
A good source of vitamin C, A, potassium, phosphorus, magnesium, sodium and calcium.

Curries:
Stimulating spice. High antioxidant and anti carcinogenic and reduces prostate cancer. Rich in vitamin A, K, E, beta carotene, folate, potassium, calcium, phosphorus, magnesium, manganese and sodium.

Eels:
Any of various snakelike fish. High in vitamin A and D.

Eggs:
Plain, raw chicken eggs enhance libido and balances hormone levels. High source of vitamin B6, B5, D, folate, choline, beta carotene, phosphorus, potassium, calcium, selenium, magnesium, iron and zinc.

Fennel:
Aromatic seed of an Eurasian plant. An ancient Egyptian aphrodisiac. Source of natural plant estrogens.

Figs:
A sweet , hollow, pear-shaped fruit of trees or shrubs of the genus Ficus. Traditionally used as sexual stimulant.

Fish:
A good source of fat soluble vitamins A, D, B12, B1, B2, B6, E, thiamine, riboflavin and pyridoxine.

Flesh:
A type of reptile of suborder Sauria or lacertilia..

Garlic:
Is said to stimulate sex desires. Contains vitamin A, C and D.

Ginger:
Has a soothing properties, and is an stimulant to the circulatory system. A tropical perennial that grows from an aromatic, tuberous rhizome. A good source of vitamin C.

Ginseng:
Any of several plants of the genus Panax. According to ancient Chinese philosophy it helps to restore potency in men due to its blood circulation support, and provides vitality and strength of a bull.

Honey:
Egyptian used it to cure infertility and impotence. The great Persian physician Avicenna in 11th century prescribed honey mixed with ginger and little pepper to stimulate those love hormones.

Liquorice (Licorice):
Chewing on licorice root stimulates desire particularly for women.

Lobster:
Rich in zinc, phosphorus, vitamin B12, copper and selenium.

Milk:
Very ancient sex stimulator. in Indian old tradition a mixture of milk, crushed pepper and almond, or a mixture of milk with honey, ghee (a clarified, semifluid butter), licorice (sweet root of a Mediterranean perennial plant) and sugar is uses to stimulate sex desire.

Mushrooms:
Rich in vitamin D, C niacin, pantothenic acid, potassium, phosphorus, magnesium, selenium, calcium, Sodium and iron.

Mussels:
Any of several marine bivalve mollusks, such as oyster or a clam. High in B complex and omega 3 fatty acids.

Mustard:
The seed of any various Eurasian plants of the genus Brassica. Stimulate sexual glands and increases desire. Rich in vitamin B3, selenium, tryptophan, omega 3 fatty acids, phosphorus, magnesium, manganese, dietary fiber, iron, calcium and zinc.

Onion:
Was considered potent aphrodisiacs by ancient Romans and Greeks. A good source of vitamin C, folate, potassium, phosphorus, calcium,

magnesium, sodium, and selenium.

Orange:
Rich in vitamin A, C, B1, folate, pantothenic acid, potassium, calcium, phosphorus, magnesium, and selenium.

Oyster:
High in zinc, and high in D-aspartic acid and N-methyl-D-aspartate, which increases testosterone levels.

Peach:
Rich in vitamin A, C, folate, niacin, potassium, phosphorus, calcium, magnesium, selenium, iron and manganese.

Pineapple:
Used in the homeopathic treatment for impotence. Eat with chili powder or mix with honey or rum. Rich in vitamin C, A, folate, potassium, magnesium, calcium and phosphorus.

Pine Nuts:
High in zinc, which is necessary for sperm production. Rich in vitamin E, A, K, niacin, folate, potassium, phosphorus, magnesium, calcium, manganese zinc and iron.

Pistachio:
Rich in vitamin A, folate, potassium, phosphorus, magnesium, calcium, sodium, iron and selenium.

Pumpkin Seeds:
High in amino acids and boosts energy. Rich in vitamin A, folate, potassium, magnesium, phosphorus, calcium, sodium, zinc and iron.

Sage (Salvia officinal):
Leaves of any plants of the genus Salvia. Has aromatic grayish-green leaves used as a cooking herb. Rich in vitamin A, C, B-complex, calcium and potassium.

Strawberries:
Considered to be the fruit of love. Rich in vitamin A, C, folate,

potassium, phosphorus, calcium, magnesium, selenium, iron and manganese.

Sweet Basil:
An old world aromatic annual herb in the mint family. Stimulate the sex drive and boost fertility.

Truffles:
Any various fleshy edible fungi. Believed to contain a chemical similar to humans' sex hormones.

Turnips:
An ancient Greeks and Romans aphrodisiac.

Vanilla:
The scent of vanilla stimulate both male and female libido.

Wasabi (Horseradish):
Super spicy green stuff that usually comes with Sushi. A good source of vitamin A, beta carotene, C, B6, folate, potassium, calcium, magnesium, phosphorus, sodium and zinc.

Wine:
Relaxes and helps to stimulate our senses. In moderation amount, other wise has opposite effect.

Coffee:
Stimulate both body and the mind. In moderation amount, other wise has opposite effect.

ANAPHRODISIACS
Anti Aphrodisiacs
"based on folklore"

Tobacco, Dill, Lentil, Lettuce, Watercress, Rue, Water Lily, excess of Alcohol, Cocaine and Ecstasy (MDMA).

VITAMINS and MINERALS
(Essential vitamins and minerals for a healthy sexual function)

(Consult your physician before taking any of these supplements)

Vitamin A:
Essential for the production of sex hormones like estrogen and testosterone. Regulates sexual growth, development and reproduction.

B Group Vitamins (B1, B2, B3, B5, B6, B12, Folate):
Regulate sex hormone function and testosterone levels. Decreases production of prolactin, a hormone that reduces sex drive.

Vitamin B2 (niacin):
Enhances penile circulation by enlarging blood vessels. Stimulates discharge of histamine, needed for orgasm.

Vitamin C:
Increases semen volume and boost sex drive.

Vitamin E:
Protects sex hormones from oxidation and degradation. Helps prevent prostatitis (inflammation of prostate gland).

Zinc:
Essential for male sexual maturity and fertility. Increases sperm production and boosts sex drive.

Thiamin, Sodium, Magnesium, Phosphorus, Potassium, Iron, Copper, Calcium, Riboflavin, Niacin, Folic Acid, Biotin, Pantothenic Acid, Bromelain, Chromium, Molybdenum, Selenium, Manganese, Boron.

HERBS
(Essential herbs to induce sexual activity)

**(These herbs might be hazardous for some people.
Consult your physician before taking any of these herbs)**

Asafetida: An Indian dried, powdered herb used as a sexual stimulant in Ayurvedic medicine.

Asian Red Ginseng - Panax Ginseng: Improves erectile function, sexual desire, and intercourse satisfaction. It is an antioxidant, and anticancer.

Avena Sativa Extract (Oats): Increases testosterone such as tribulus terrestris.

Catuaba Bark Extract: Used for sexual weakness, nervousness and poor memory.

Cuscuta Seed Extract: Has positive effects on sperm health and motility, and invigorates the reproductive system. Has a high content of flavonoids and has strong antioxidant properties.

Damiana Extract: A potent aphrodisiac, which is an agent that stimulates sexual desire.

Epimedium Leaf Extract: Enhances male and female libido and sexual performance.

Ginkgo Biloba Leaf: Antioxidant, circulation and memory enhancing.

Gladiolus Root: Boosts sexual health.

Grape Seed Extract: Powerful anti-oxidants.

Hawthorn Berry - Fructus Crataegi: Both the Greeks and Romans used to associate it with marriage & fertility. Enhances enzyme metabolism and oxygen utilization in the heart muscle.

Kava Kava: Anti anxiety and sleep enhancing. A sedative, muscle relaxant, and effective for nervousness and insomnia. The relaxed state caused by the herb contributes to aphrodisiac effect.

L-arginine (Nitric oxide 'NO'): Improves immune function and reduces wound-healing time. Increases sexual performance and helps to maintain erection.

Lycopene: Antioxidant found in tomatoes for a healthy prostate.

Maca: Sold as "natural Viagra"..

Muira Puama: An Amazonian aphrodisiac.

Orchid Bulbs: Boosts sexual health.

Peruvian Maca Root: Increases energy and stamina.

Saw Palmetto Berry Extract: For a healthy prostate.

Siberian Ginseng Root: Anti-stress, stamina increase,

St. John's Wort: Anti depression.

Stinging Nettle extract: For a healthy prostate.

Tribulus Terrestris Extract: Sold as "natural Viagra".

Valerian: Relaxing and inducing deep sleep.

Velvet Deer Antler: Oriental medicine to treat male impotence.

Yohimbe: Sold as "natural Viagra", may help erection.

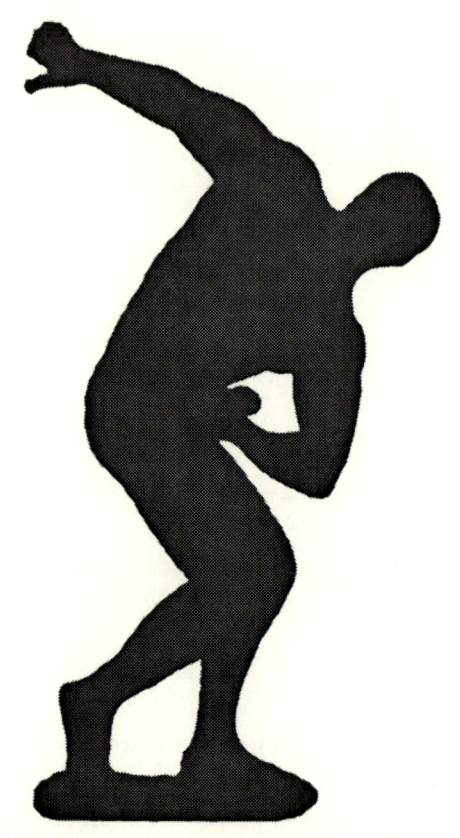

Fitness by Penis

Section 1

Stand-up Non-lubricated Exercises

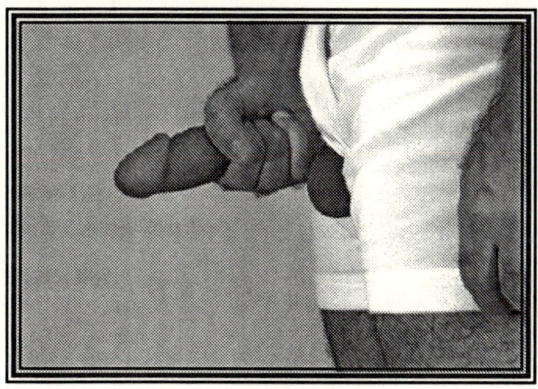

1- <u>Warm-up Fist Exercise</u>

Penis state: Semi erect
Target muscles: Hand, Fingers
Penis strengths: Warm-up, Thickness
Safety: "Warm-up exercise" Be gentle with squeezing.
Repeat: 15 times each position

Stand straight with legs slightly apart.

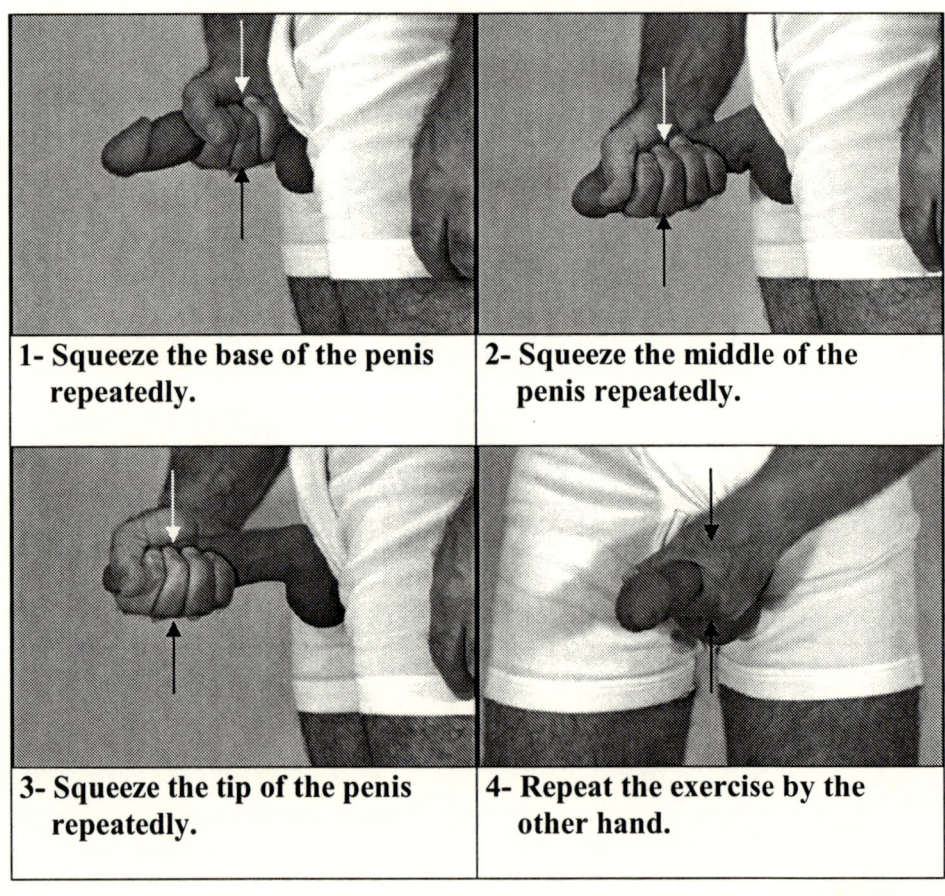

1- Squeeze the base of the penis repeatedly.	2- Squeeze the middle of the penis repeatedly.
3- Squeeze the tip of the penis repeatedly.	4- Repeat the exercise by the other hand.

2- <u>Warm-up Shoulder Pull</u>

Penis state: Flaccid
Target muscles: Back shoulder, Chest
Penis strengths: Warm-up, Length increase
Safety: "Warm-up exercise" Start with gentle pulls.
Repeat: 50 times

Stand straight with legs slightly apart.

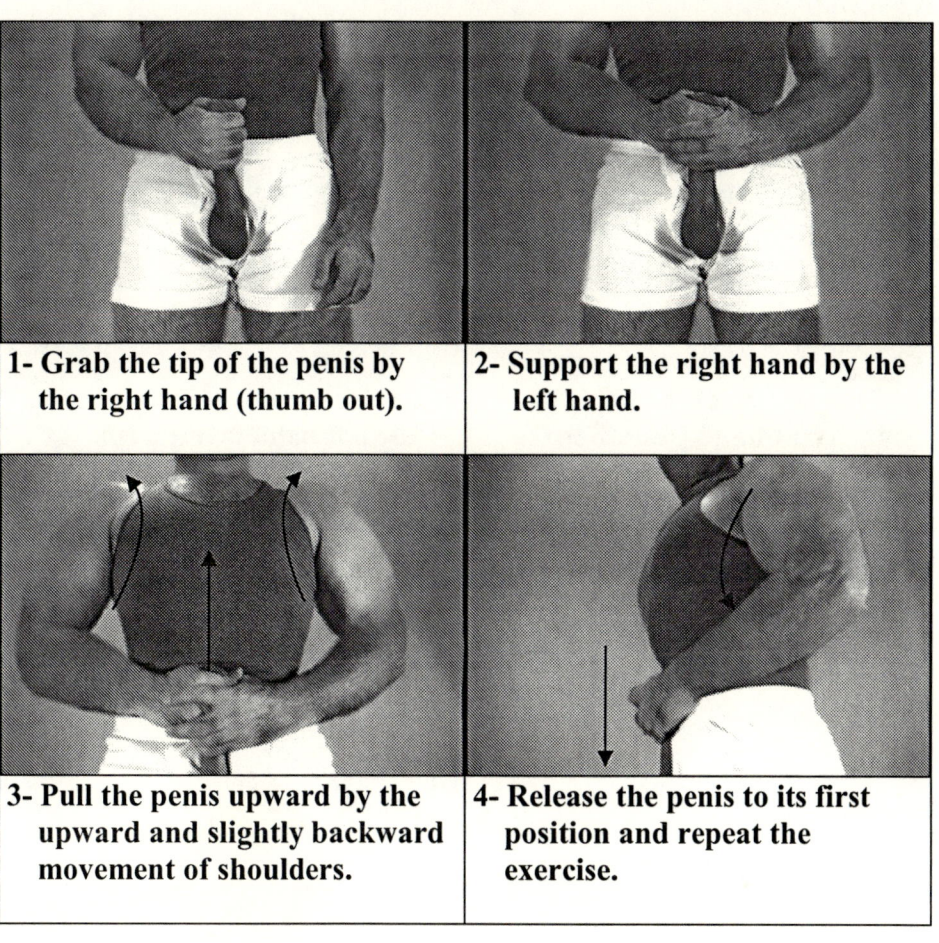

1- Grab the tip of the penis by the right hand (thumb out).	2- Support the right hand by the left hand.
3- Pull the penis upward by the upward and slightly backward movement of shoulders.	4- Release the penis to its first position and repeat the exercise.

3- <u>Up and Down</u>

Penis state: Flaccid
Target muscles: Chest, Arm, Forearm
Penis strengths: Base stretch, Length increase
Safety: Do not put pressure on the lower back.
Repeat: 50 times

Stand straight with legs slightly apart, and then lean slightly forward from your waist.

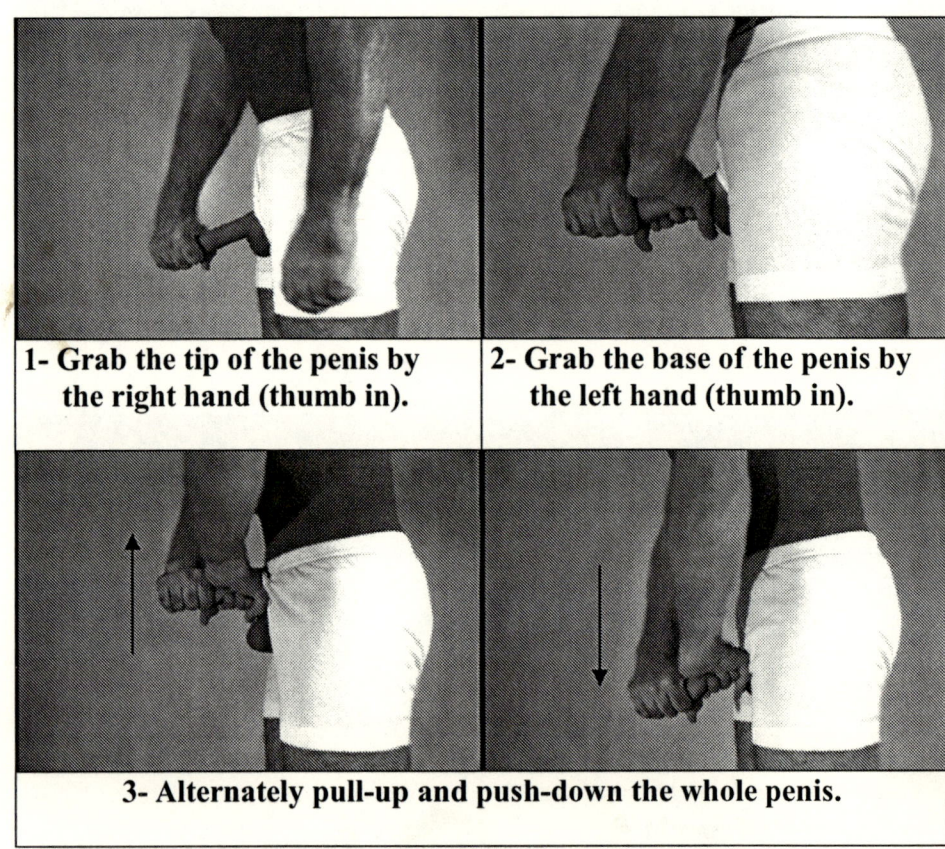

1- Grab the tip of the penis by the right hand (thumb in).	**2- Grab the base of the penis by the left hand (thumb in).**

3- Alternately pull-up and push-down the whole penis.

4- <u>Vertical Circular Movement</u>

Penis state: Flaccid
Target muscles: Chest, Arm, Forearm
Penis strengths: Base stretch, Length increase
Safety: Do not put pressure on the lower back..
Repeat: 25 times clockwise, 25 times counter clockwise

Stand straight with legs slightly apart, and then lean slightly forward from your waist.

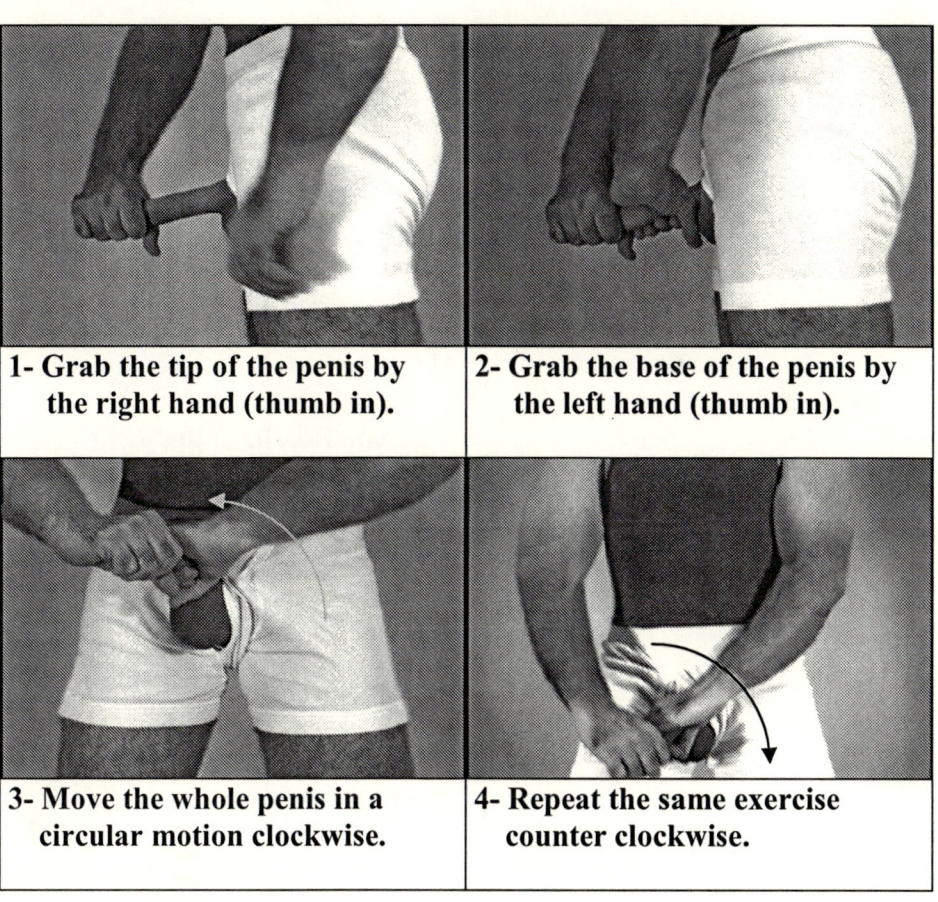

1- Grab the tip of the penis by the right hand (thumb in).	2- Grab the base of the penis by the left hand (thumb in).
3- Move the whole penis in a circular motion clockwise.	4- Repeat the same exercise counter clockwise.

5- <u>Horizontal Circular Movement</u>

Penis state: Flaccid
Target muscles: Chest, Arm, Forearm
Penis strengths: Base stretch, Length increase
Safety: Do not put pressure on the lower back..
Repeat: 25 times clockwise, 25 times counter clockwise

Stand with legs apart then bend your knees and slightly lean forward from your waist.

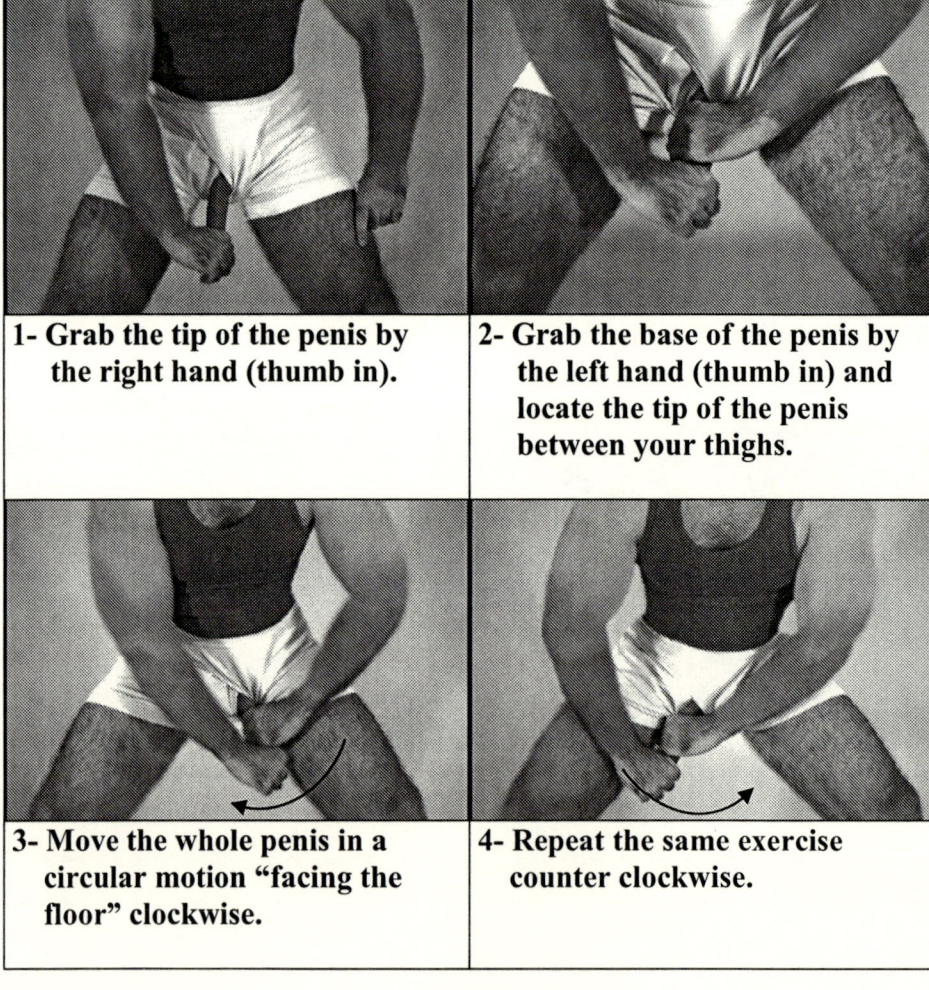

1- Grab the tip of the penis by the right hand (thumb in).	2- Grab the base of the penis by the left hand (thumb in) and locate the tip of the penis between your thighs.
3- Move the whole penis in a circular motion "facing the floor" clockwise.	4- Repeat the same exercise counter clockwise.

6- Shoulder Twist

Penis state: Flaccid
Target muscles: Shoulder, Chest, Abdominal
Penis strengths: Base, Length increase
Safety: Be gentle with your waist.
Repeat: 25 times

Stand straight with legs slightly apart.

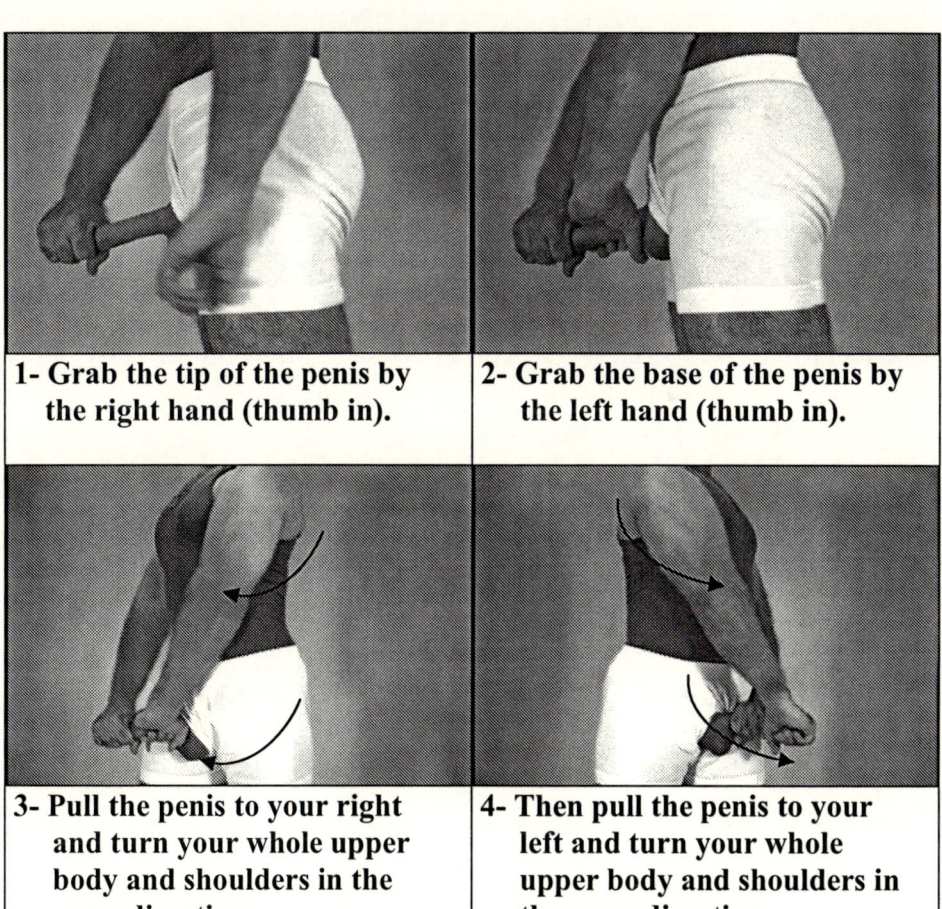

1- Grab the tip of the penis by the right hand (thumb in).	2- Grab the base of the penis by the left hand (thumb in).
3- Pull the penis to your right and turn your whole upper body and shoulders in the same direction.	4- Then pull the penis to your left and turn your whole upper body and shoulders in the same direction.

7- <u>Waist Twist</u>

Penis state: Flaccid
Target muscles: Waist, Abdominal
Penis strengths: Base, Length increase
Safety: Be gentle with your waist.
Repeat: 25 times

Stand straight with legs slightly apart.

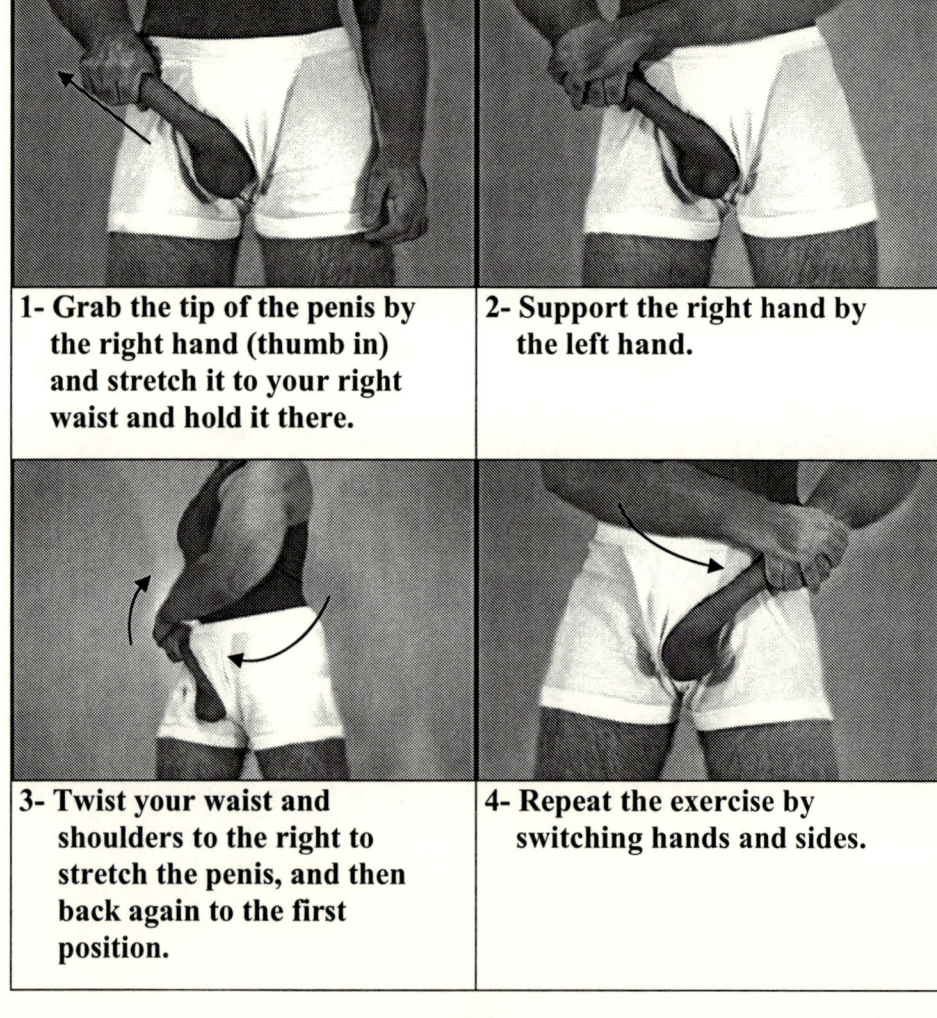

1- Grab the tip of the penis by the right hand (thumb in) and stretch it to your right waist and hold it there.

2- Support the right hand by the left hand.

3- Twist your waist and shoulders to the right to stretch the penis, and then back again to the first position.

4- Repeat the exercise by switching hands and sides.

8- <u>Multiple Pull</u>

Penis state: Flaccid
Target muscles: Forearm, Arm, Side chest, Wrist
Penis strengths: Length increase
Safety: Avoid harsh pulling.
Repeat: 20 times

Stand straight with legs slightly apart.

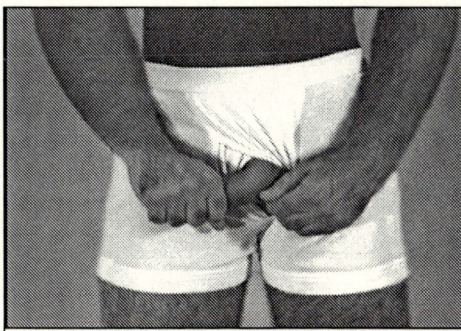	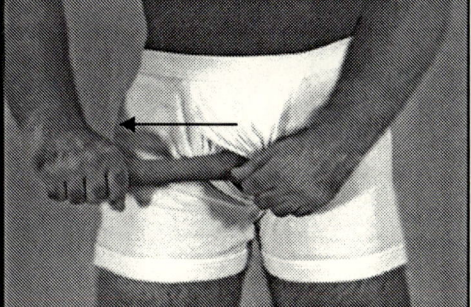
1- Grab the tip of the penis by the right hand (thumb in) and support your testicles from dangling by your left hand.	**2- Pull and stroke the whole penis sideway toward your right waist and then return to the first position.**

Repeat also the same exercise in the following directions;

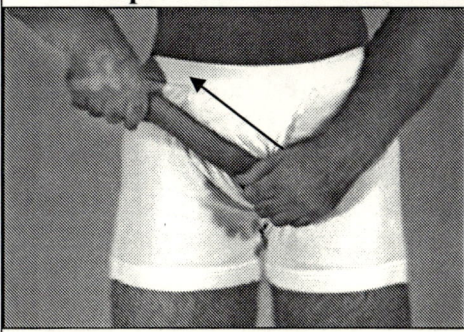	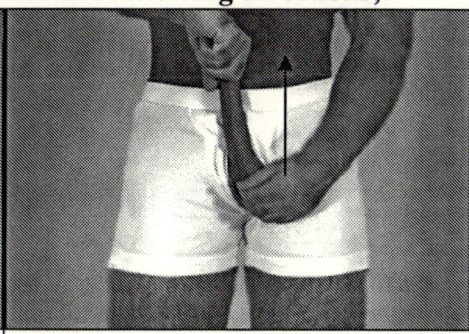
***** **Pull upward toward your right armpit.**	***** **Pull upward toward your head.**

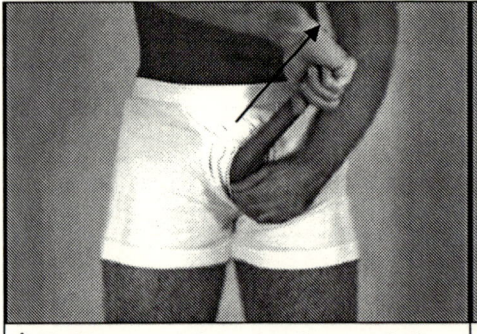

* **Pull upward toward your left armpit.**

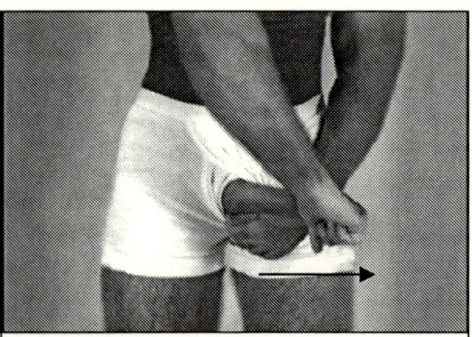

* **Pull sideway toward your left waist.**

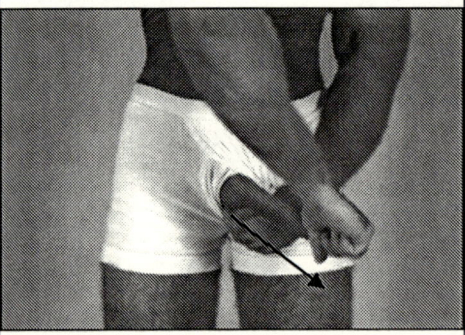

* **Pull downward toward your left knee**

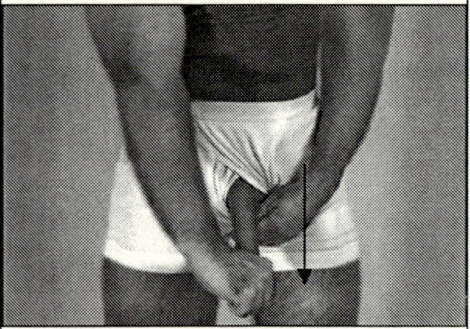

* **Pull downward between your thighs.**

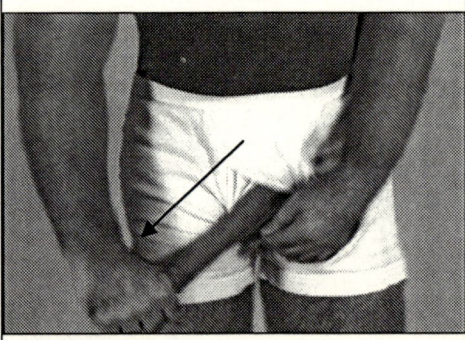

* **Pull downward toward your right knee.**

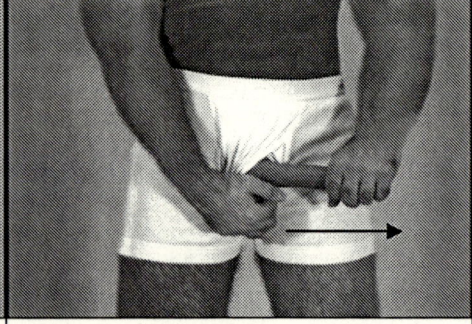

Then repeat all the exercises by your left hand.

9- In and Out

Penis state: Flaccid
Target muscles: Arm, Chest
Penis strengths: Length increase
Safety: Be gentle with strokes.
Repeat: 50 times

Stand straight with legs slightly apart.

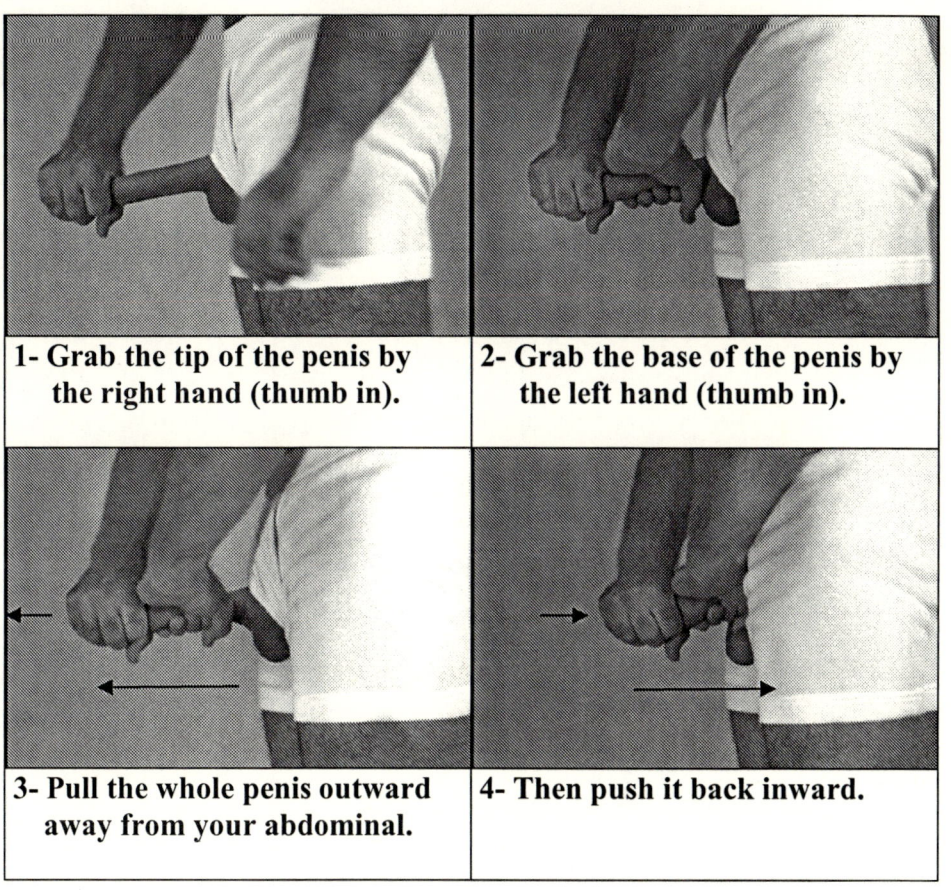

1- Grab the tip of the penis by the right hand (thumb in).	2- Grab the base of the penis by the left hand (thumb in).
3- Pull the whole penis outward away from your abdominal.	4- Then push it back inward.

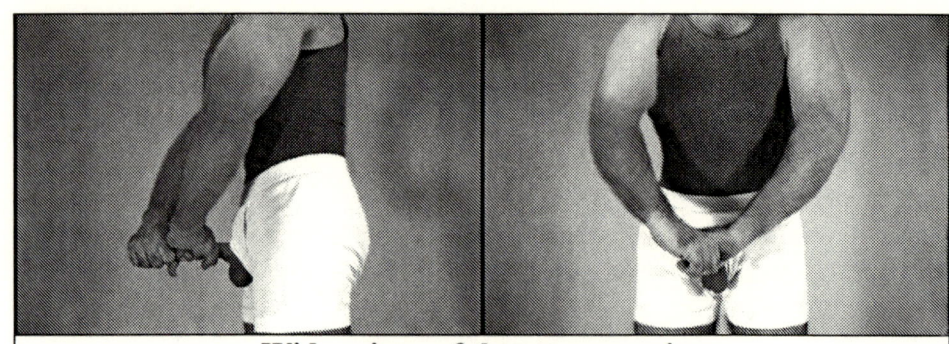

Wider views of the same exercise

10- <u>Under Leg</u>

Penis state: Flaccid
Target muscles: Thigh, Arm
Penis strengths: Length increase
Safety: Be careful not to put too much pressure on the penis.
       Maintain a balance by supporting your body.
Repeat: 50 times

Stand straight with legs slightly apart.

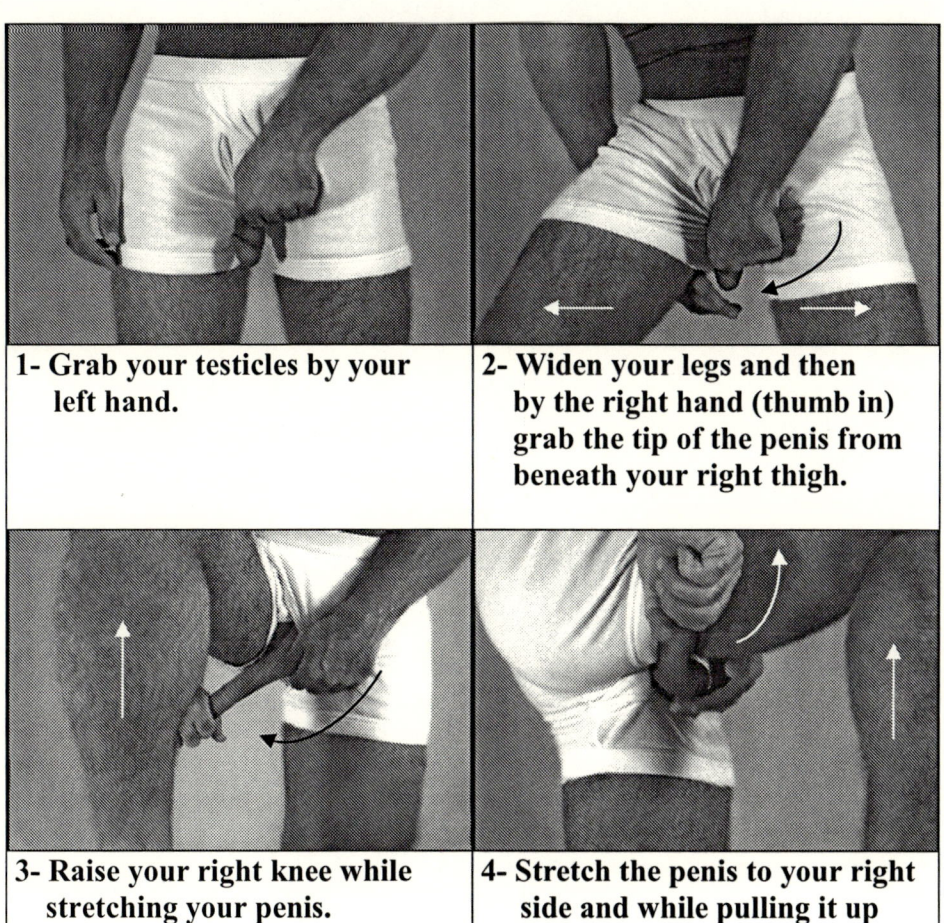

1- Grab your testicles by your left hand.	**2- Widen your legs and then by the right hand (thumb in) grab the tip of the penis from beneath your right thigh.**
3- Raise your right knee while stretching your penis.	**4- Stretch the penis to your right side and while pulling it up hold it there.**

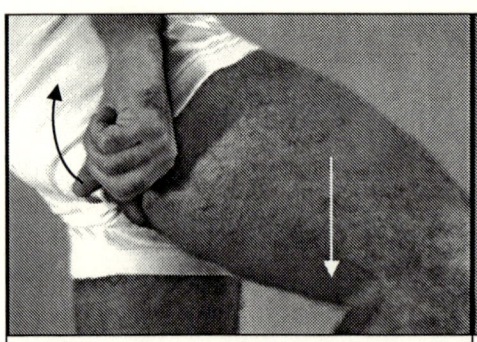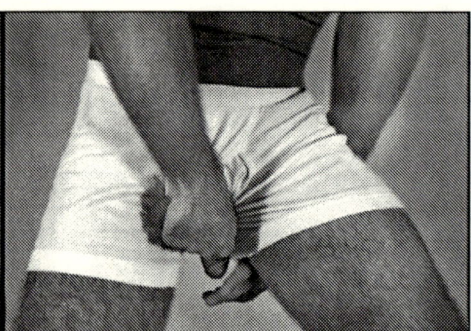

5-Then, alternately push your leg over the penis and then pull it back.	Repeat the same exercise with your left leg and left hand.

11- <u>Over Leg</u>

Penis state: Flaccid
Target muscles: Thigh, Arm
Penis strengths: Length increase
Safety: Maintain a balance by supporting your body.
Repeat: 50 times

Stand straight with legs slightly apart.

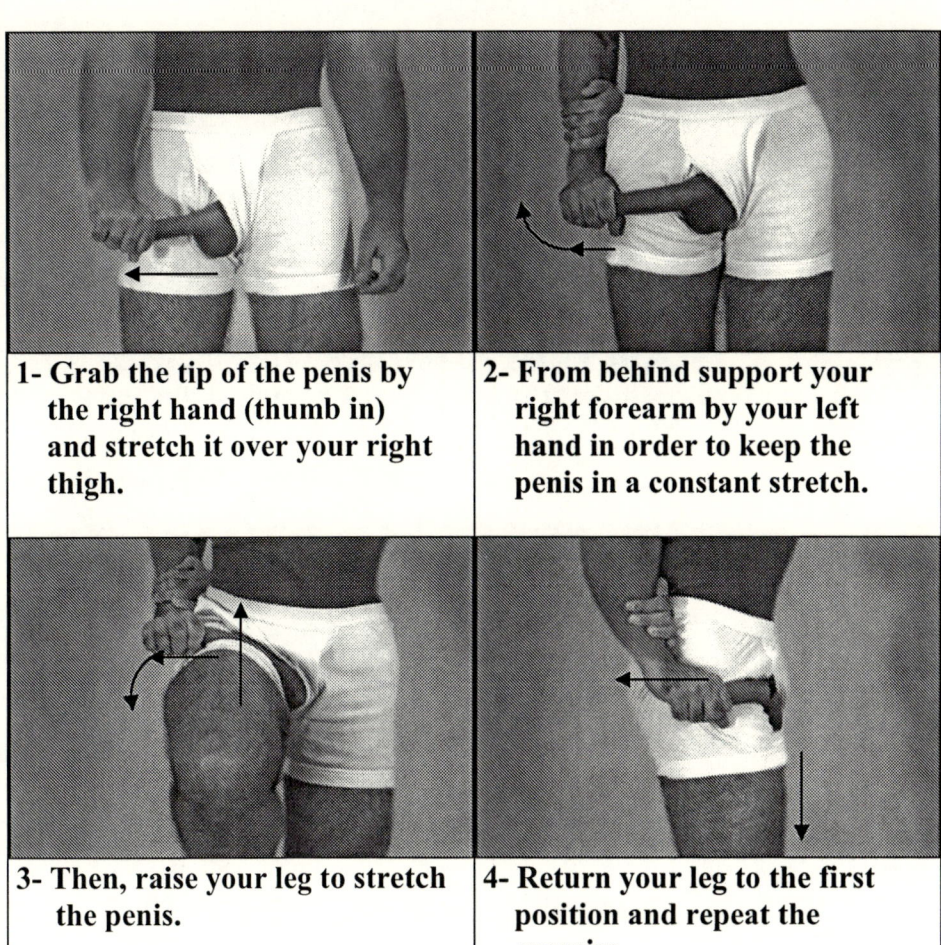

1- Grab the tip of the penis by the right hand (thumb in) and stretch it over your right thigh.	2- From behind support your right forearm by your left hand in order to keep the penis in a constant stretch.
3- Then, raise your leg to stretch the penis.	4- Return your leg to the first position and repeat the exercise.

Repeat the same exercise with your left leg and left hand.

12- __Both Hands Back Pull__

Penis state: Flaccid
Target muscles: Upper back, Arm, Side chest
Penis strengths: Length increase
Safety: Be careful not to put pressure on testicles.
Repeat: 50 times

Stand straight with legs slightly apart.

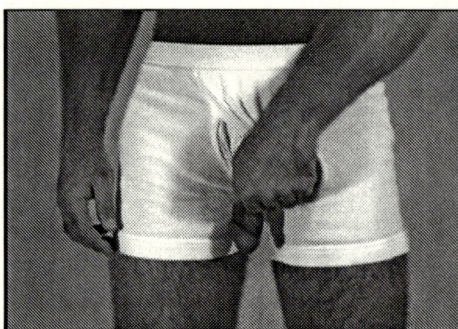

1- Grab your testicles by your left hand.

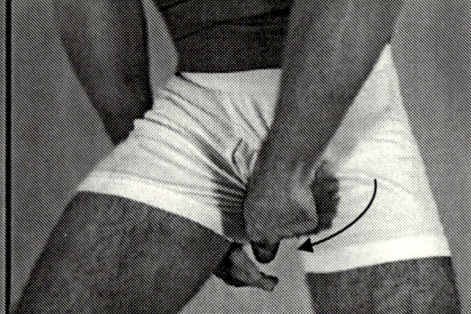

2- By your thumb guide the tip of the penis toward the back to your right hand.

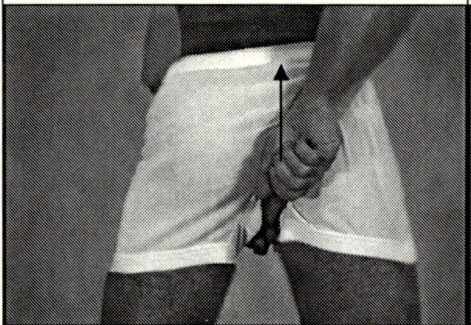

3- By the right hand grab the tip of the penis from behind and stretch it up.

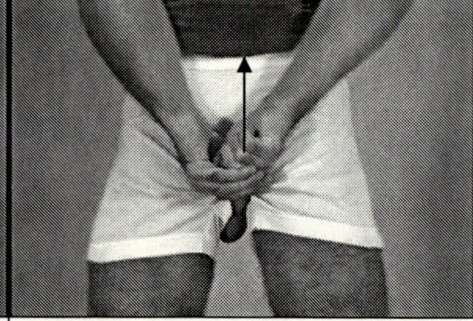

4- Release your testicles and with your left hand support your right hand from behind.

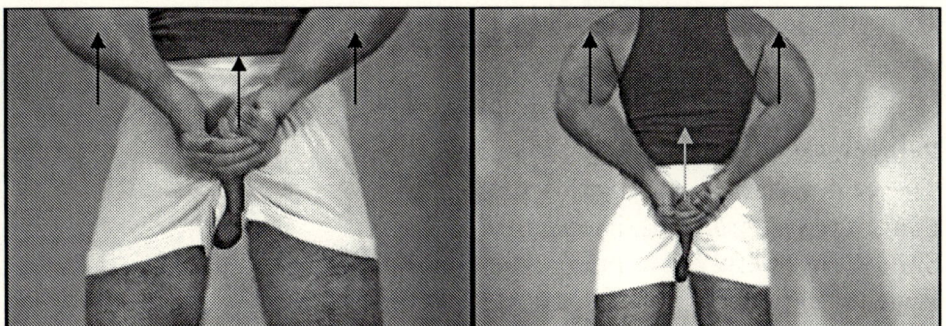

5- Then by both hands and the force of shoulders and forearms stretch and pull the penis upward and then return it to the first position.

13- <u>One Hand Back Pull</u>

Penis state: Flaccid
Target muscles: Upper back, Arm, Side chest
Penis strengths: Length increase
Safety: Be careful not to put pressure on testicles.
Repeat: 30 times

Stand straight with legs slightly apart.

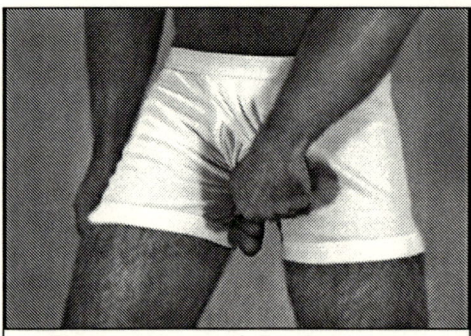	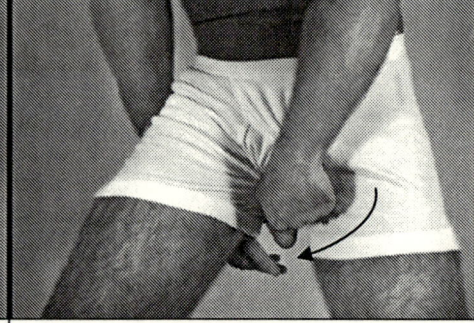
1- Grab your testicles by your left hand.	2- By your thumb guide the tip of the penis toward the back to your right hand.
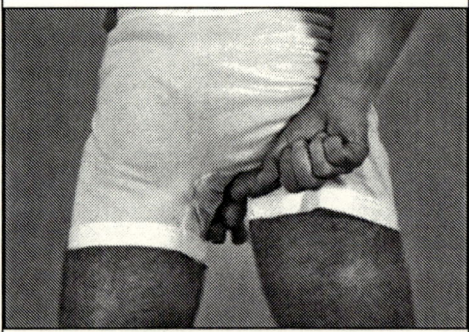	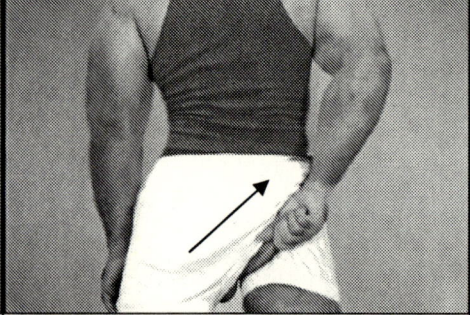
3- By the right hand grab the tip of the penis from behind and then release your testicles.	4- Stretch the penis upward toward your right waist and then return it to the first position.
Repeat the same exercise with your left hand in the opposite direction.	

14- <u>Bend Stretch – A</u>

Penis state: Flaccid
Target muscles: Back leg, Waist
Penis strengths: Length increase
Safety: Do not over stretch the penis.
Repeat: One minute

Stand straight with legs slightly apart.

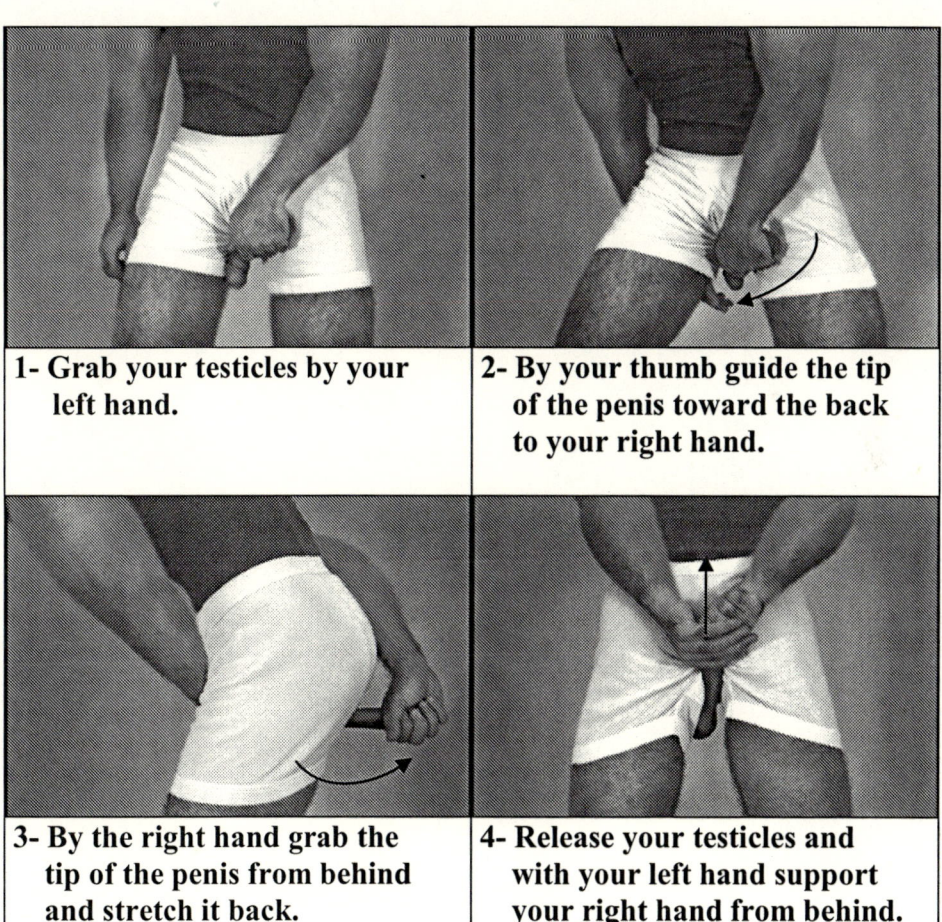

1- Grab your testicles by your left hand.	2- By your thumb guide the tip of the penis toward the back to your right hand.
3- By the right hand grab the tip of the penis from behind and stretch it back.	4- Release your testicles and with your left hand support your right hand from behind.

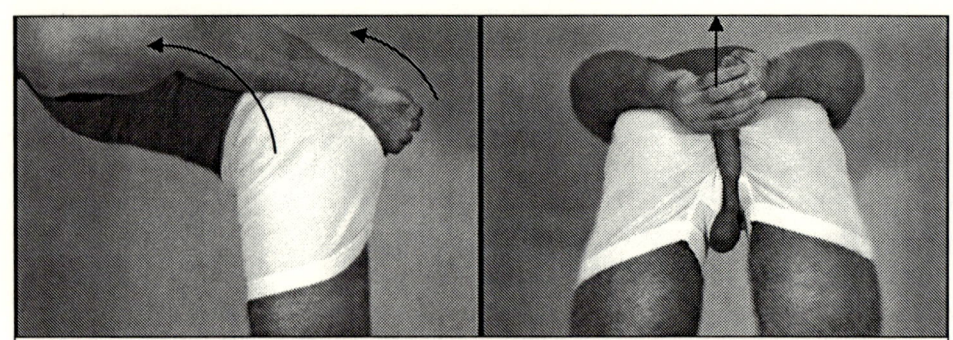

5- Bend forward halfway to stretch the penis and hold it there.

15- <u>Bend Stretch – B</u>

Penis state: Flaccid
Target muscles: Back leg, Waist
Penis strengths: Base stretch, Length increase
Safety: Do not put pressure on the lower back.
Repeat: 25 times

Stand with legs slightly apart then bend your knees and slightly lean forward from your waist.

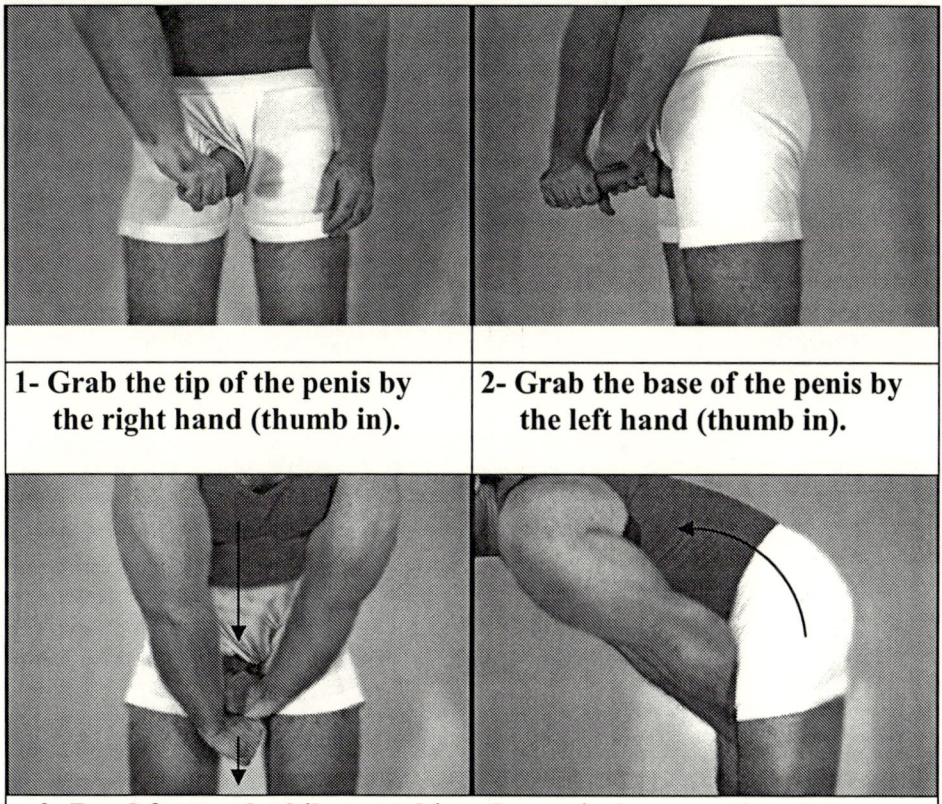

| 1- Grab the tip of the penis by the right hand (thumb in). | 2- Grab the base of the penis by the left hand (thumb in). |

3- Bend forward while stretching the penis downward and then return to the first position.

16- Foot Workout

Penis state: Flaccid
Target muscles: Foot, Calf
Penis strengths: Length increase
Safety: Be careful not to push hard on testicles.
Repeat: 30 times

Stand straight with legs slightly apart.

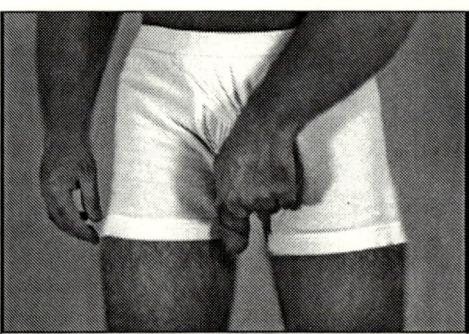

1- Grab your testicles by your left hand.

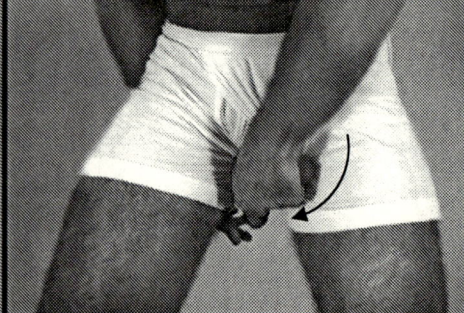

2- By your thumb guide the tip of the penis toward the back to your right hand.

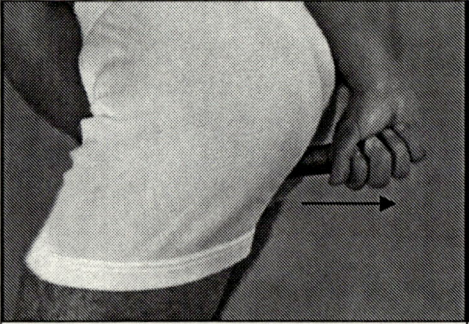

3- By the right hand grab the tip of the penis from behind and stretch it back.

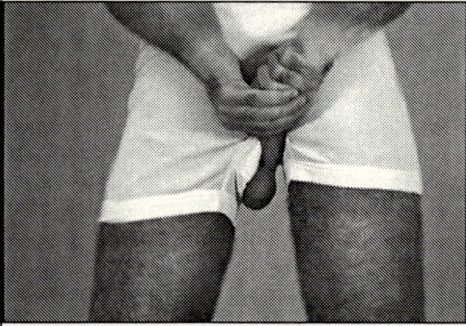

4- Release your testicles and with your left hand support your right hand from behind.

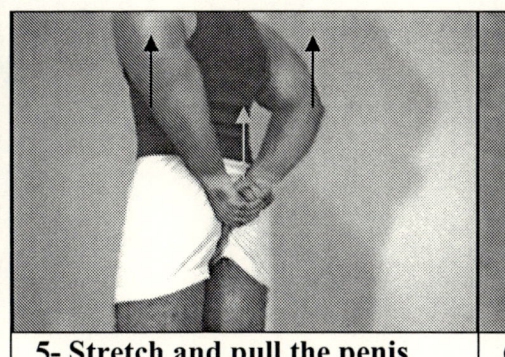	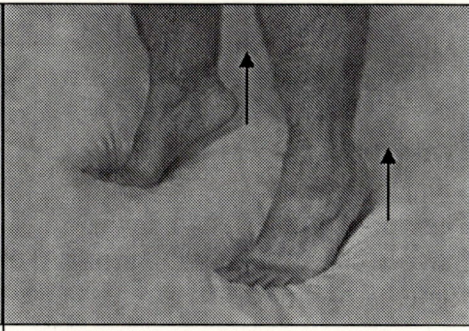
5- Stretch and pull the penis upward and hold it there.	**6- Raise and lower your heels alternately and with each upward motion of your body stretch your penis upward.**

17- <u>Legs Workout</u>

Penis state: Flaccid
Target muscles: Leg, Knee
Penis strengths: Length increase
Safety: Be careful not to push hard on testicles.
Repeat: 40 times

Stand straight with legs slightly apart

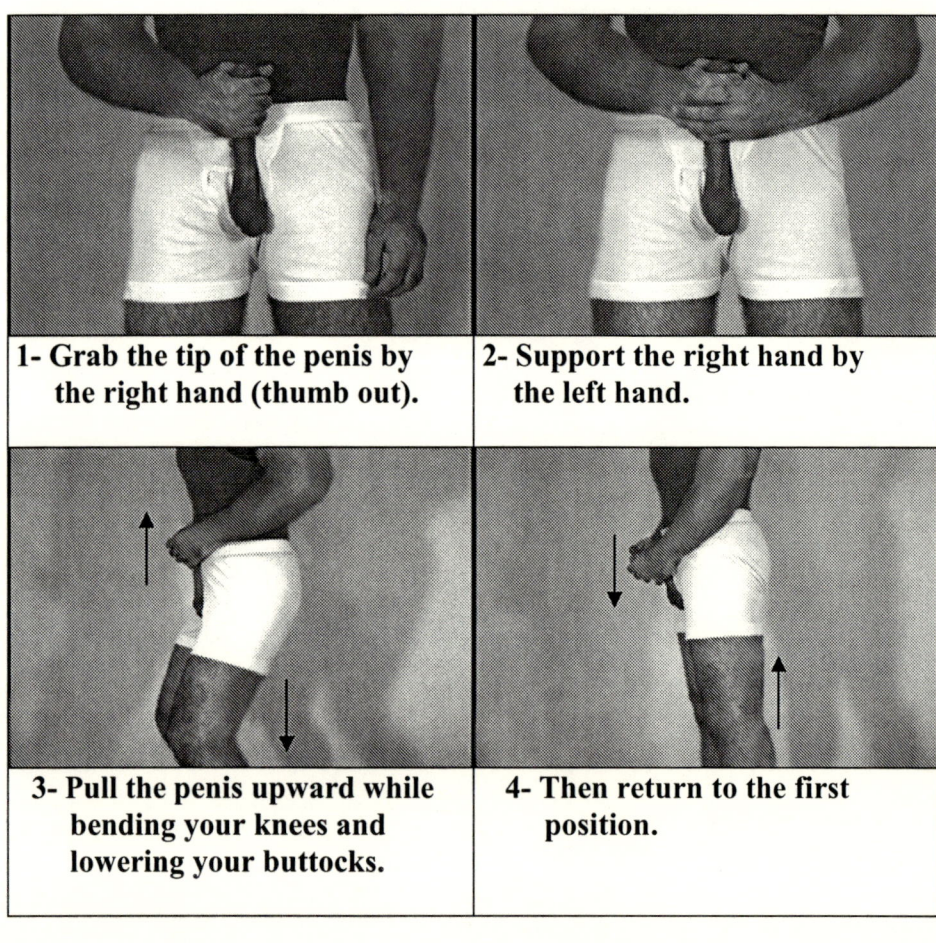

1- Grab the tip of the penis by the right hand (thumb out).	**2- Support the right hand by the left hand.**
3- Pull the penis upward while bending your knees and lowering your buttocks.	**4- Then return to the first position.**

18- Bend Pull

Penis state: Flaccid
Target muscles: Forearm, Arm. Armpit
Penis strengths: Length increase
Safety: Support your back
Repeat: 20 times each

Bend half way from your waist while supporting your body by your left hand against a bar or a chair.

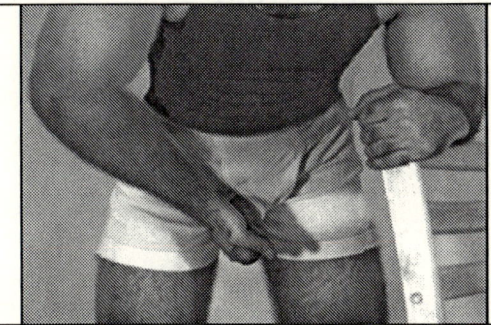

1- Grab the penis from the middle by the right hand (thumb out)

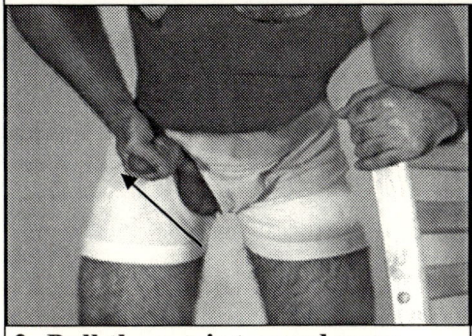 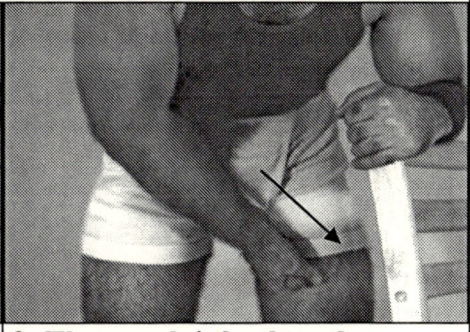

| **2- Pull the penis toward your right shoulder and arm.** | **3- Then push it back to the opposite direction toward your left leg.** |

Repeat also the same exercise in the following directions;

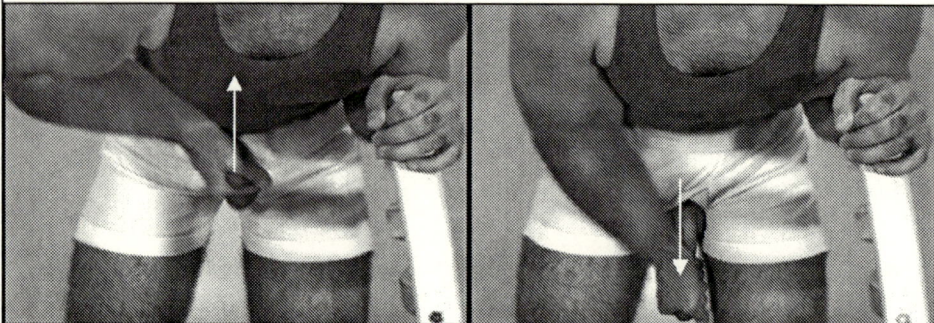

* Pull it toward your head and then push it to the opposite direction.

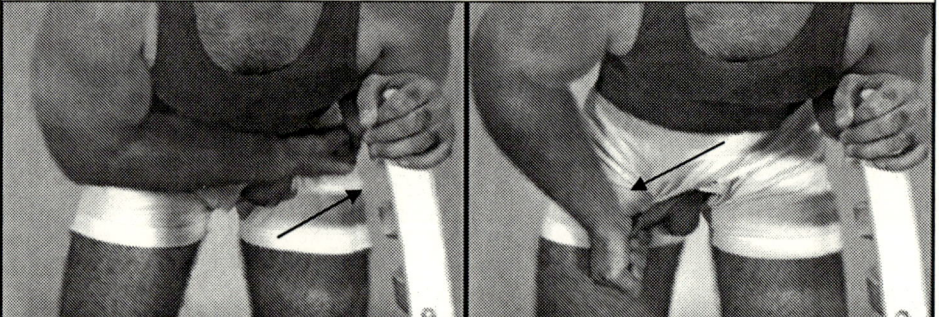

* Pull it toward your left shoulder and push it to the opposite direction.

Repeat the whole exercises by your left hand.

19- Side Stretch – A

Penis state: Flaccid
Target muscles: Side
Penis strengths: Length increase
Safety: Be gentle with your side and avoid over stretching the penis.
Repeat: 30 times

Stand straight with legs slightly apart.

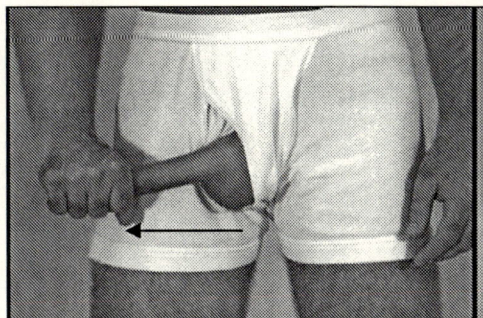

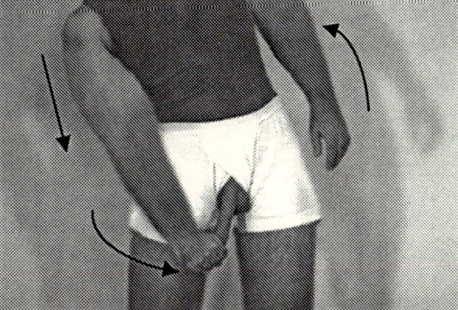

1- Grab the tip of the penis by the right hand (thumb in) and stretch it to your right side.	2- While keeping the penis stretched and keeping your hand straight bend from your waits toward your right side.

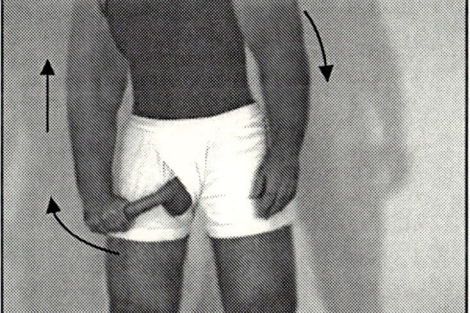

3- Then return to the first position.

Repeat the whole exercise by your left hand in the opposite direction.

20- Side Stretch – B

Penis state: Flaccid
Target muscles: Side
Penis strengths: Length increase
Safety: Be gentle with your side and avoid over stretching the penis.
Repeat: 30 times

Stand straight with legs slightly apart.

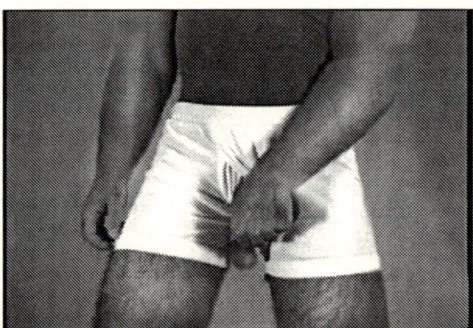

1- Grab your testicles by your left hand.

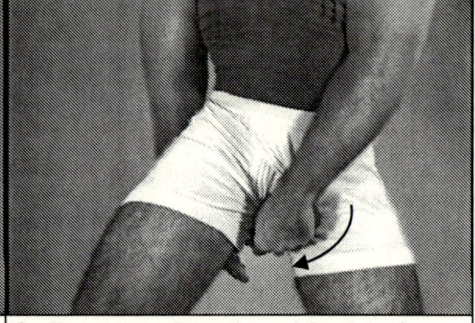

2- By your thumb guide the tip of the penis toward the back to your right hand.

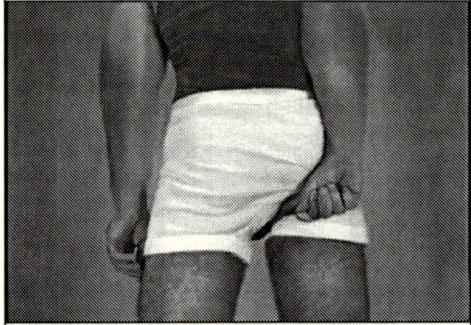

3- By the right hand grab the tip of the penis from behind and then release your testicles.

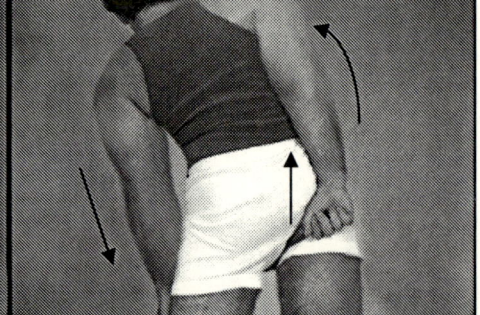

4- While holding the penis, bend sideway to your left to stretch the penis and your right side, and then return to the first position.

Repeat the whole exercise by your left hand in the opposite direction.

21- <u>Twist Stretch</u>

Penis state: Flaccid
Target muscles: Side, Waist
Penis strengths: Length increase
Safety: Be gentle with your sides, and avoid over stretching the penis.
Repeat: 30 times

Stand straight with legs slightly apart.

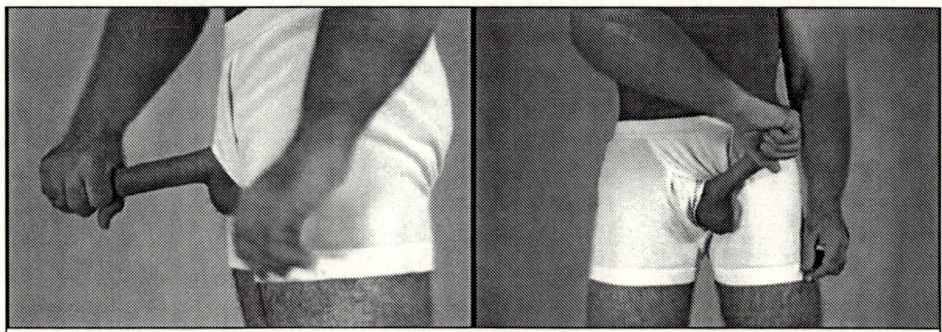

1- Grab the tip of the penis by the right hand (thumb in).

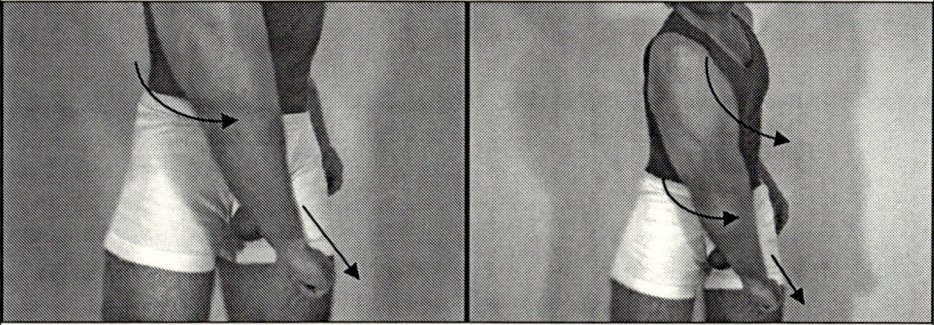

2- While keeping the penis stretched and keeping your hand straight bend from your waist toward your left knee, and then return to the first position.

Repeat the whole exercise by your left hand in the opposite direction.

22- Gear Pull

Penis state: Flaccid
Target muscles: Arm, Chest
Penis strengths: Length increase
Safety: Start with light pulling.
Repeat: 30 times

Stand straight with legs slightly apart.

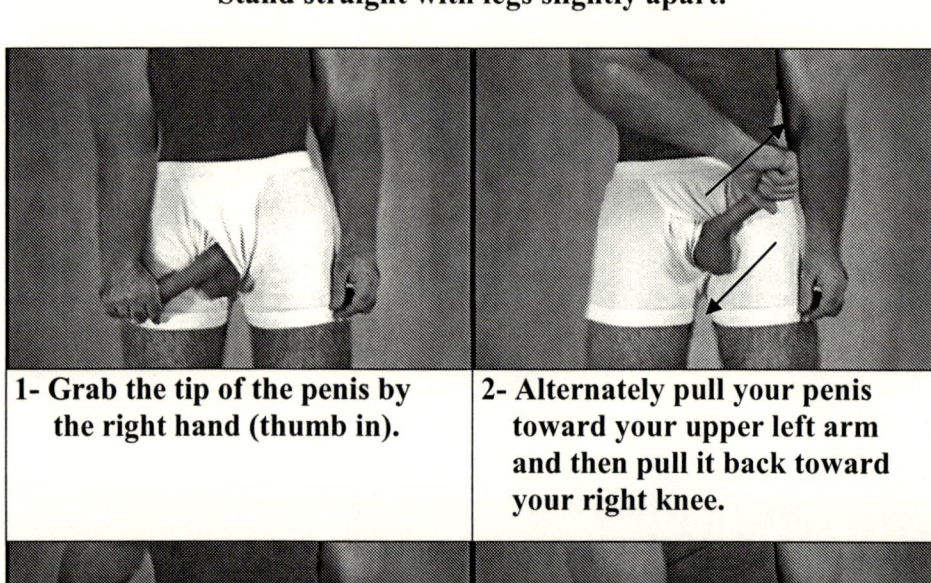

1- Grab the tip of the penis by the right hand (thumb in).	2- Alternately pull your penis toward your upper left arm and then pull it back toward your right knee.

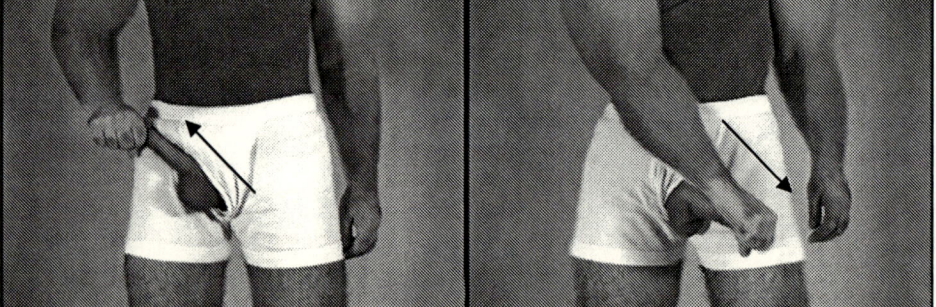

3- Repeat the same exercise in the opposite direction pulling the penis toward your upper right arm and then pull it back toward your left knee.

Repeat the whole exercise by your left hand in the opposite direction.

23- <u>Rolling Exercise</u>

Penis state: Erect
Target muscles: Forearm, arm
Penis strengths: Thickness
Safety: Roll the penis gently.
Repeat: 50 times

Stand straight with legs slightly apart.

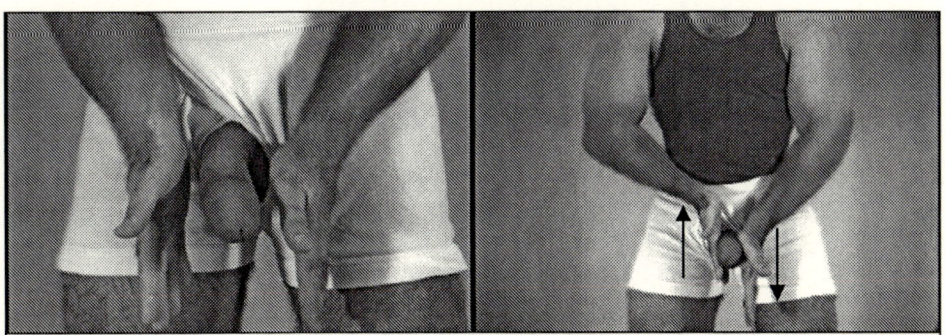

Roll your penis gently back and forth between the palms of your both hands.

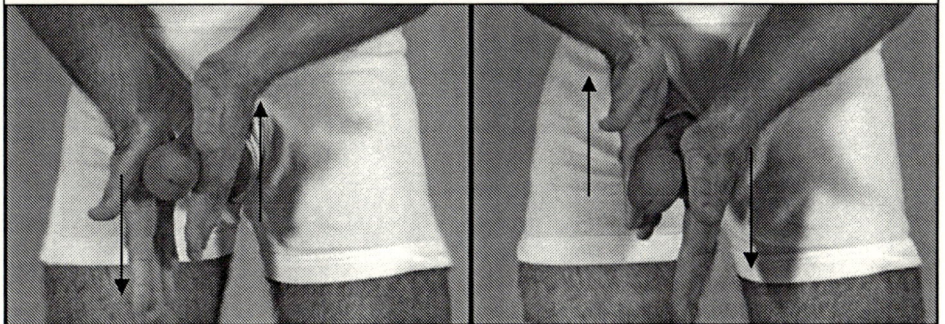

24- <u>Spinning Exercise</u>

Penis state: Flaccid
Target muscles: Arm
Penis strengths: Base muscles
Safety: Start with light spins.
Repeat: 25 times clockwise, 25 times counter clockwise

Stand straight with legs slightly apart.

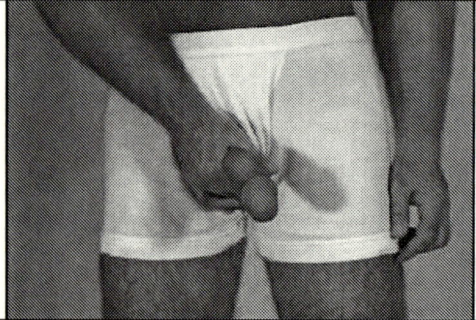

1- Grab the very base of your penis by your right hand (thumb out).

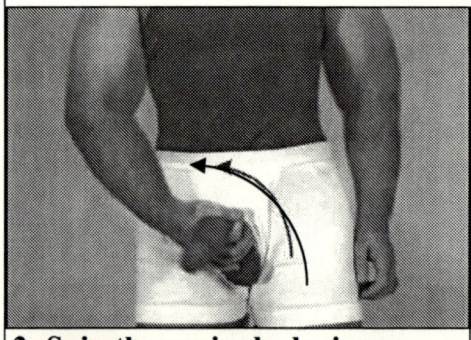

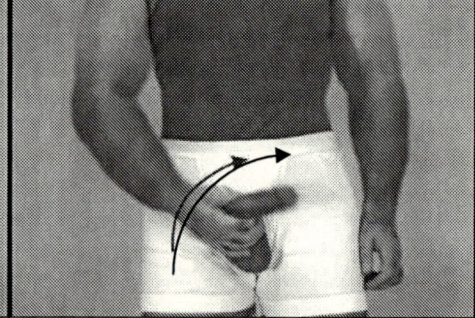

2- Spin the penis clockwise so that the tip makes the widest orbit around the center.	3- Then spin the penis counter clockwise.

Repeat the whole exercise by your left hand.

25- <u>Fold Exercise</u>

Penis state: Semi erect
Target muscles: Forearm, Wrist
Penis strengths: Middle thickness
Safety: Be very gentle with folding the penis. Start with light folding.
Repeat: 50 times

Stand straight with legs slightly apart.

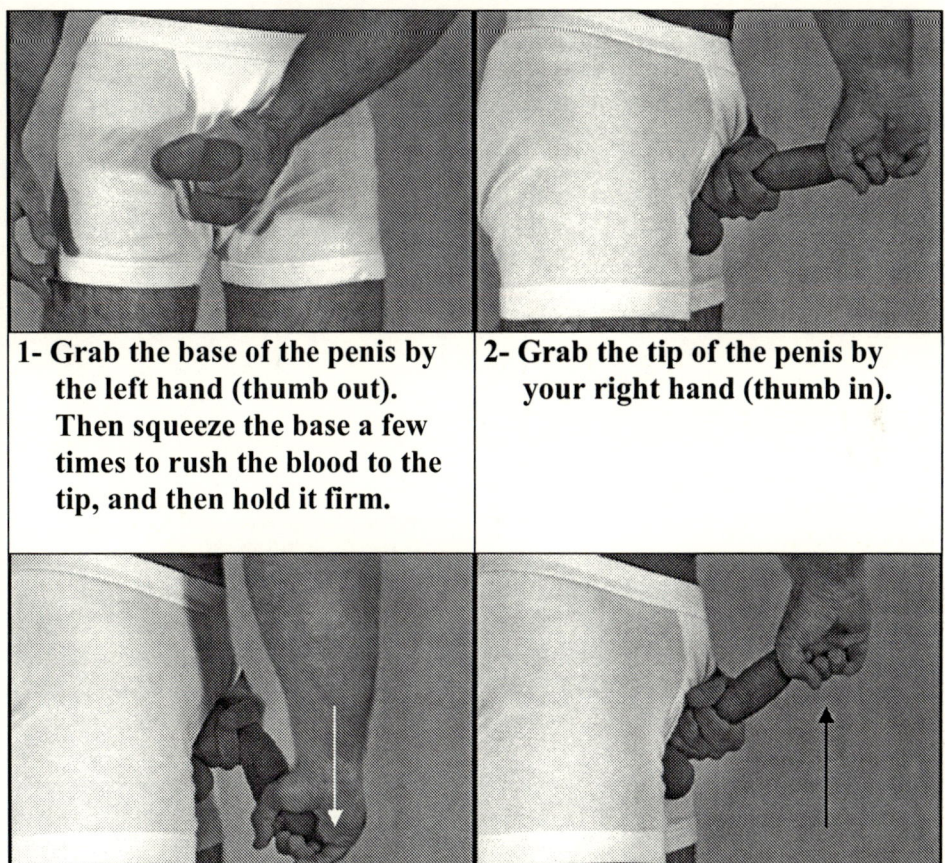

1- Grab the base of the penis by the left hand (thumb out). Then squeeze the base a few times to rush the blood to the tip, and then hold it firm.	2- Grab the tip of the penis by your right hand (thumb in).

3- Fold the penis downward and then upward alternately.

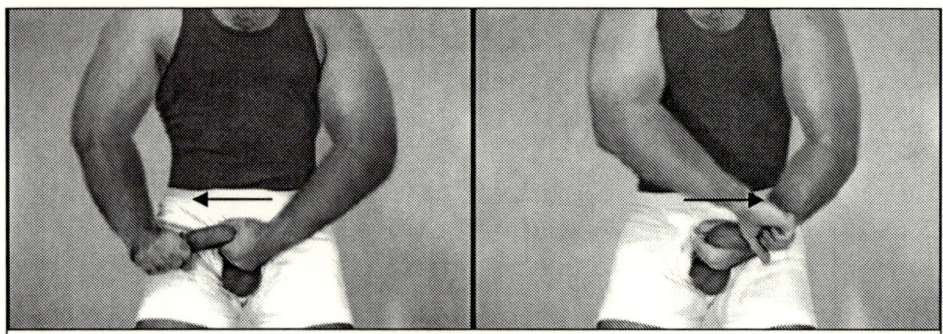

* **Repeat the same exercise by folding the penis first to your right and then to your left.**

Repeat the whole exercise by switching hands.

26- <u>Fold Fist Exercise</u>

Penis state: Flaccid
Target muscles: Hand, Wrist
Penis strengths: Thickness
Safety: Start with light squeezing.
Repeat: 25 times

Stand straight with legs slightly apart.

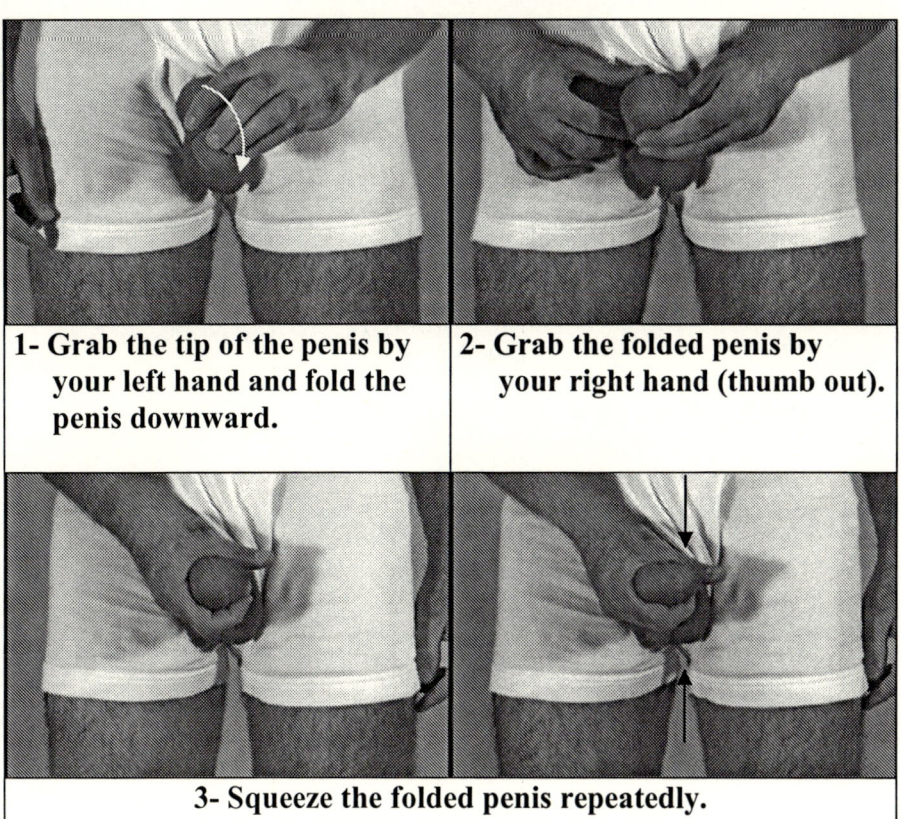

1- Grab the tip of the penis by your left hand and fold the penis downward.	2- Grab the folded penis by your right hand (thumb out).

3- Squeeze the folded penis repeatedly.

Repeat also the same exercise in the following directions;

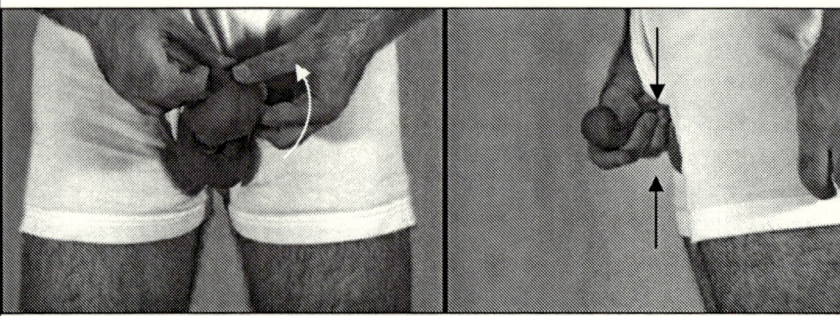

* Fold the penis upward and squeeze it repeatedly.

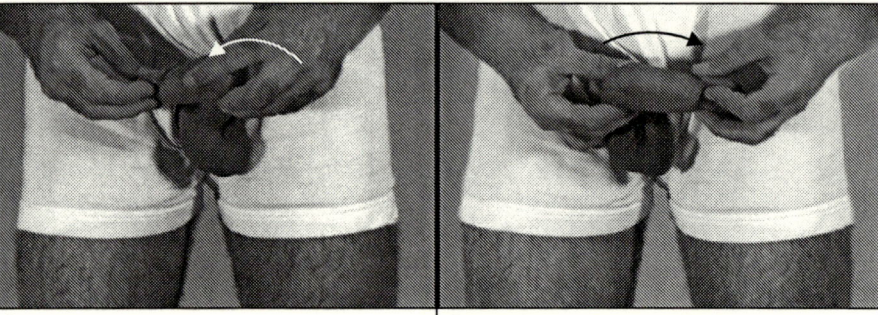

* Fold the penis sideway to your right and squeeze it repeatedly.	* Fold the penis sideway to your left and squeeze it repeatedly.

Then repeat the whole exercise by your left hand.

64

27- <u>Cross Stretch</u>

Penis state: Flaccid
Target muscles: Arm, Chest
Penis strengths: Length increase
Safety: Start with light pulling.
Repeat: 20 times

Stand straight with legs slightly apart.

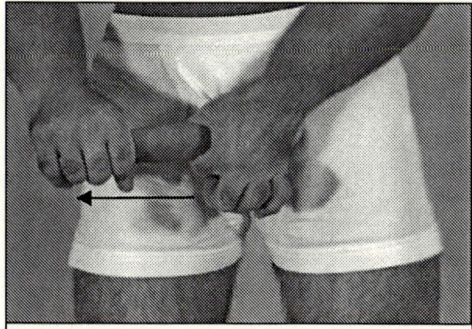 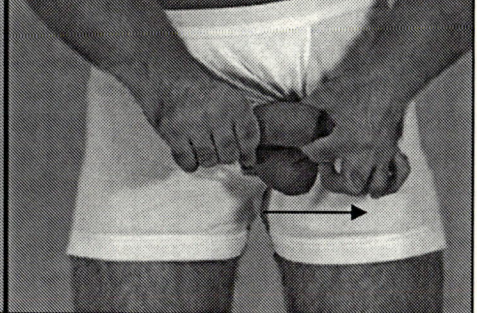

1- Grab the base of the penis by the left hand (thumb out) and then grab the tip of the penis by the right hand (thumb in) and stretch it to your right side.	2- Next by the left hand pull the base of the penis toward your left side and then return to the first position.

Repeat also the same exercise in the following directions;

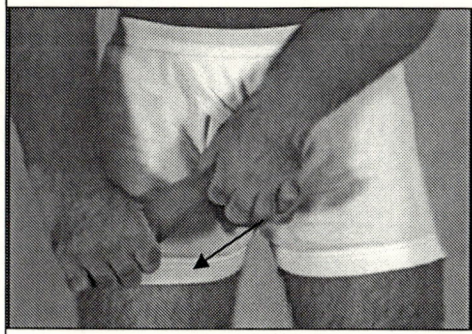 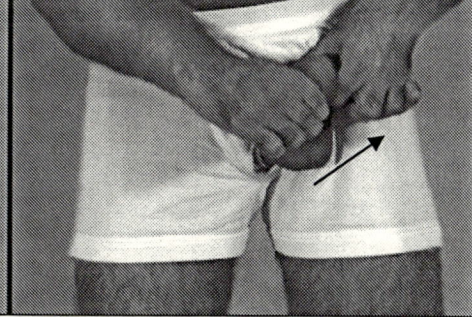

* Stretch the penis toward your right knee and then, from the base, pull it back toward your left upper arm.

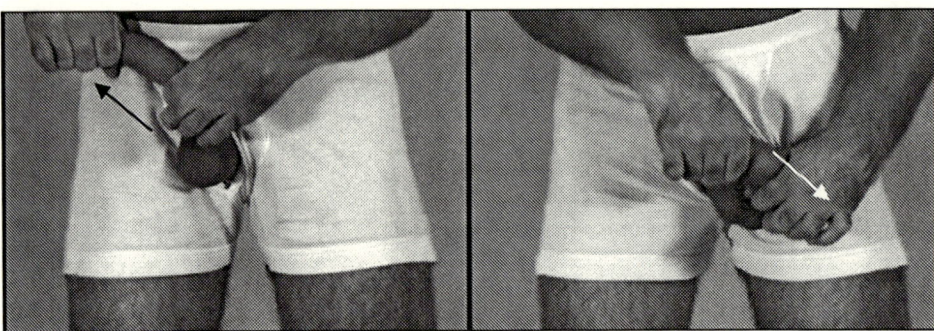

* Stretch the penis toward your right upper arm then, from the base, pull it back toward your left leg.

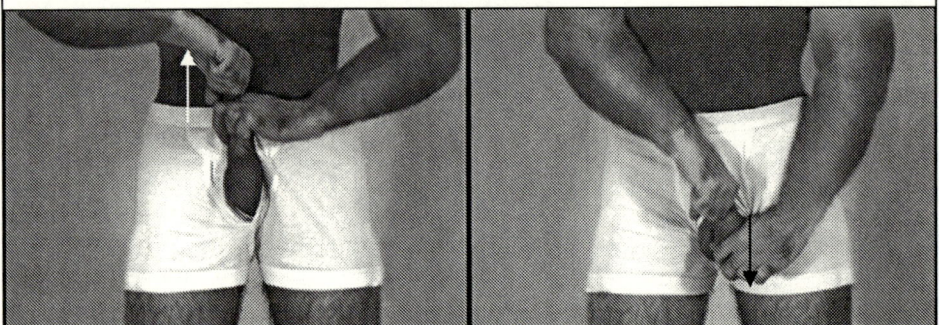

* Stretch the penis upward and then, from the base, pulling it back downward.

Repeat the whole exercise by switching hands, and pulling the penis in opposite directions.

28- <u>Crank Exercise</u>

Penis state: Erect
Target muscles: Arm, Chest
Penis strengths: Middle thickness
Safety: Be gentle with cranking, and do not exhaust the middle of penis.
Repeat: 25 times clockwise, 25 times counter clockwise

Stand straight with legs slightly apart.

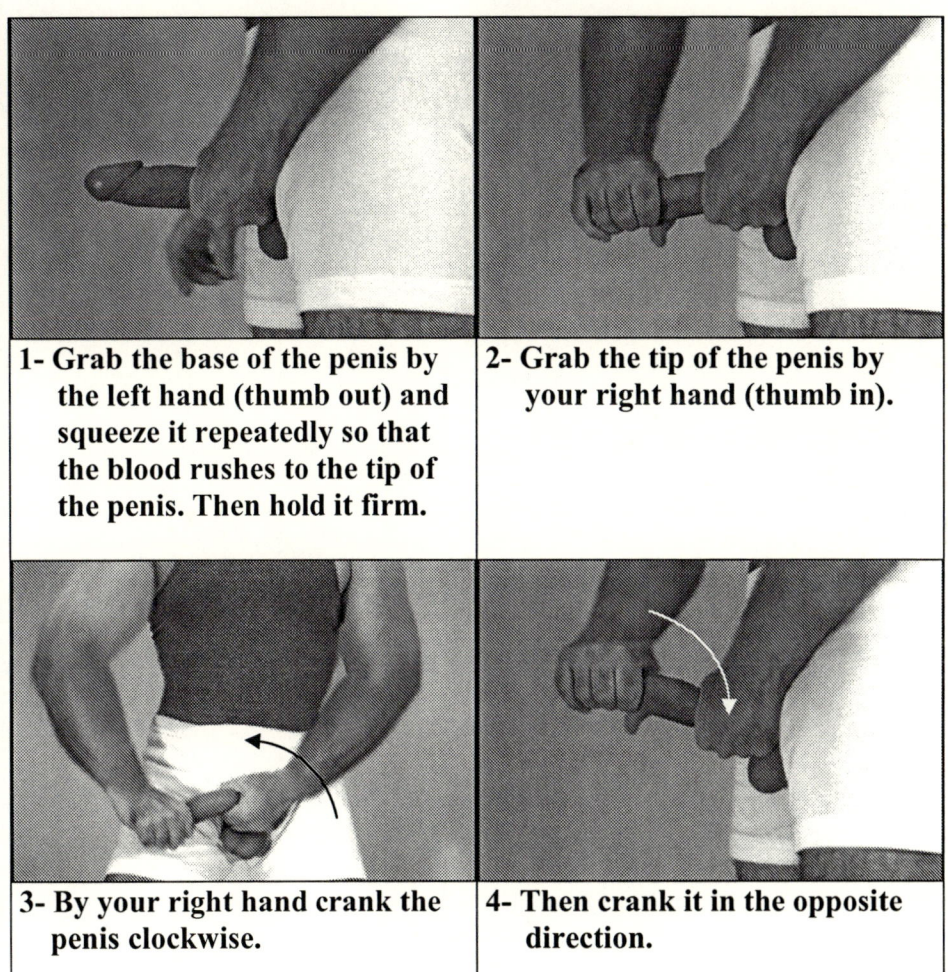

1- Grab the base of the penis by the left hand (thumb out) and squeeze it repeatedly so that the blood rushes to the tip of the penis. Then hold it firm.	2- Grab the tip of the penis by your right hand (thumb in).
3- By your right hand crank the penis clockwise.	4- Then crank it in the opposite direction.
Repeat the whole exercise by opposite hands.	

Section 2

<u>Lie-Down Non-Lubricated Exercises</u>

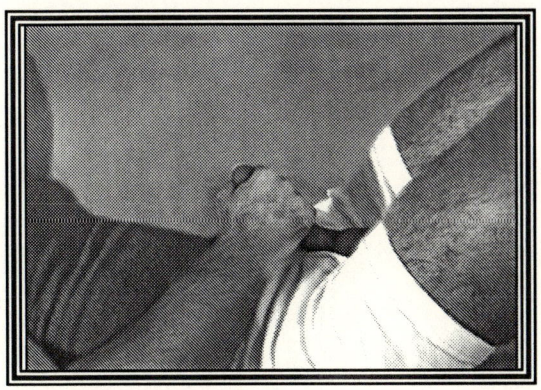

29- <u>Sit-up Stretch</u>

Penis state: Flaccid
Target muscles: Abdominal, Lower back, Arm
Penis strengths: Length increase
Safety: Support your neck by the aid of the other hand.
       Do not put your body weight on your penis.
Repeat: 30 times

Lie down on your back.

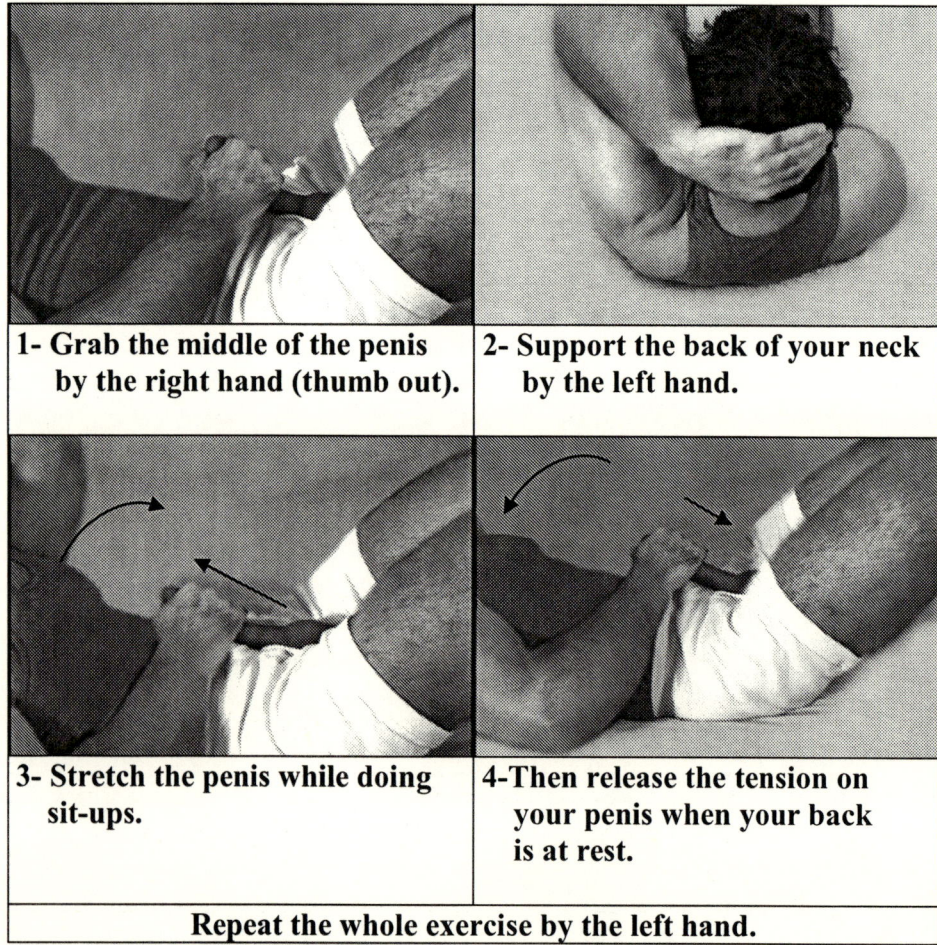

1- Grab the middle of the penis by the right hand (thumb out).	2- Support the back of your neck by the left hand.
3- Stretch the penis while doing sit-ups.	4-Then release the tension on your penis when your back is at rest.

Repeat the whole exercise by the left hand.

70

30- Leg Pull

Penis state: Flaccid
Target muscles: Thigh, Arm, Chest
Penis strengths: Length increase
Safety: Do not exceed the leg pressure over the penis.
Repeat: 30 times

Lie down on your back.

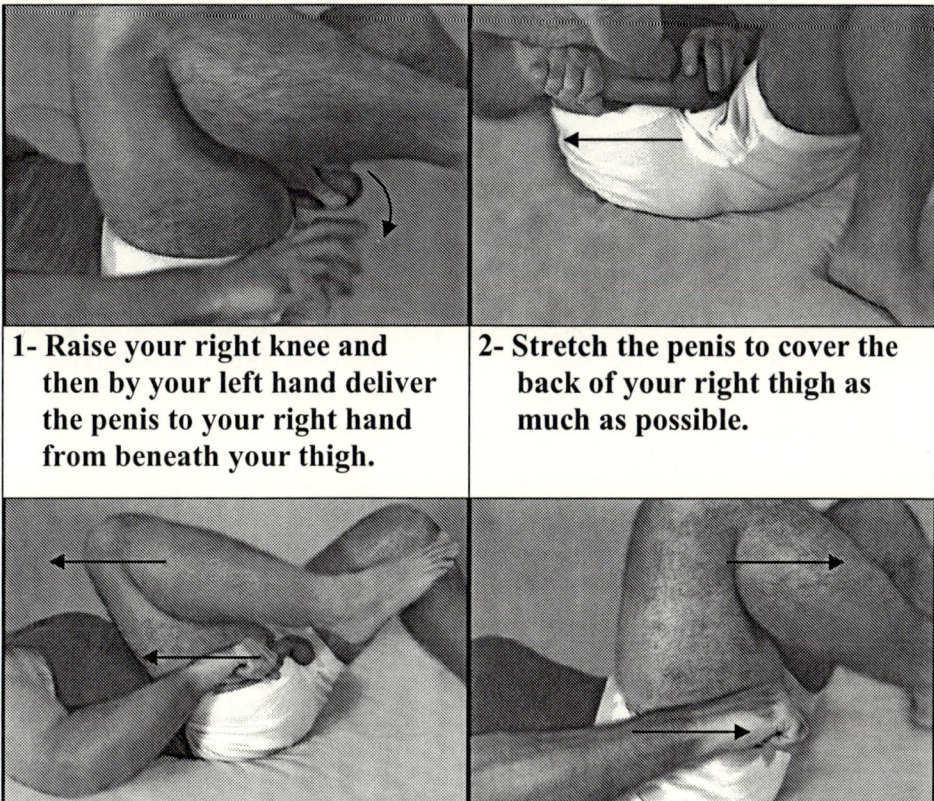

1- Raise your right knee and then by your left hand deliver the penis to your right hand from beneath your thigh.	2- Stretch the penis to cover the back of your right thigh as much as possible.

3- Then pull the penis toward your arm so that with each pull your knee moves toward your head, and then release your penis to its first position.

Repeat the whole exercise by your left hand and left leg.

31- Leg Side Pull

Penis state: Flaccid
Target muscles: Thigh, Arm
Penis strengths: Length increase
Safety: Do not exceed the leg pressure over the penis.
Repeat: 30 times

Lie down on your back.

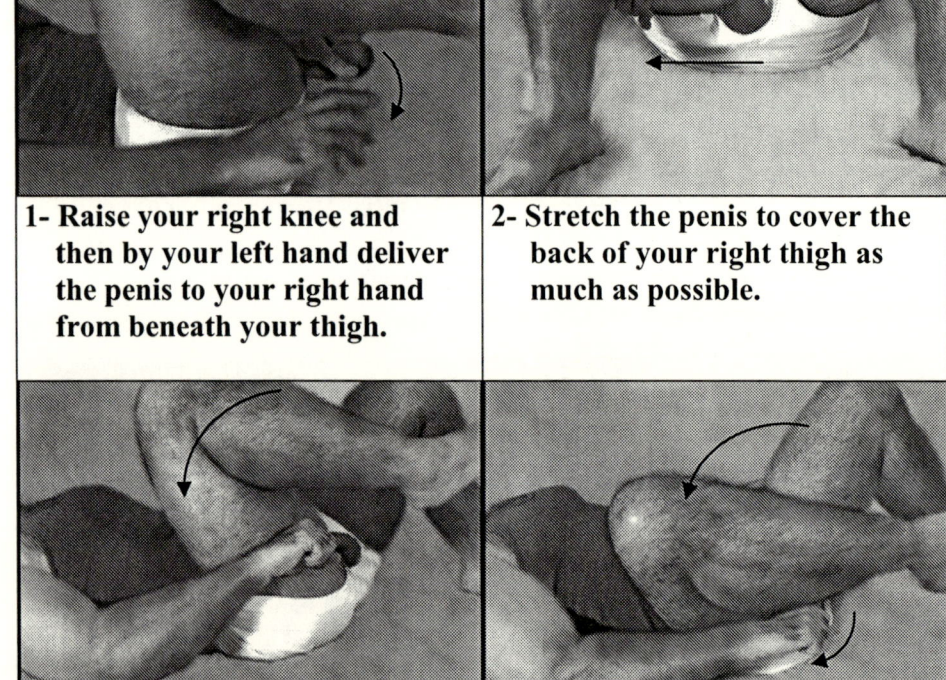

1- Raise your right knee and then by your left hand deliver the penis to your right hand from beneath your thigh.	2- Stretch the penis to cover the back of your right thigh as much as possible.

3- Then push your right knee toward your right side to stretch the penis, then release it to its original position.

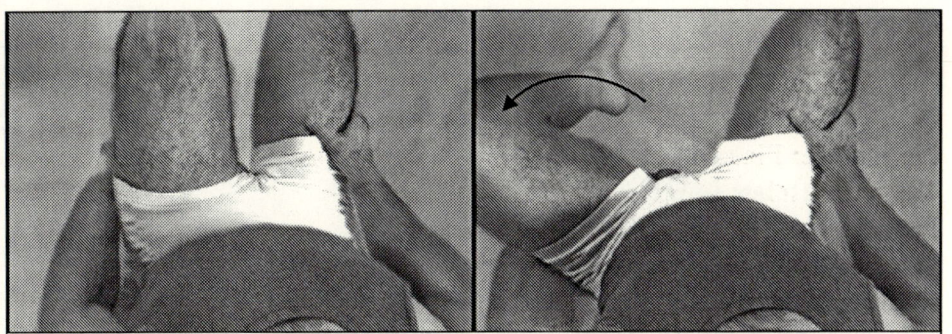

Repeat the whole exercise by your left hand and left leg.

32- <u>Lower Back Stretch</u>

Penis state: Flaccid
Target muscles: Lower back, Abdominal, Arm
Penis strengths: Length increase
Safety: Do not put too much weight on your penis.
Repeat: 30 times

Lie down on your back.

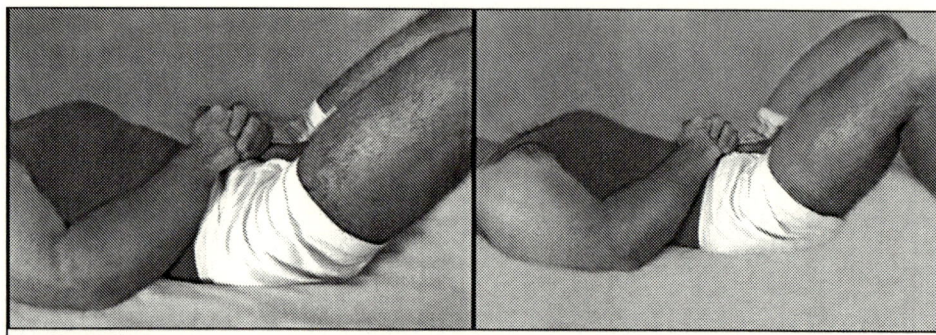

1- Bend your knees and then by both hands grab the penis from the middle.

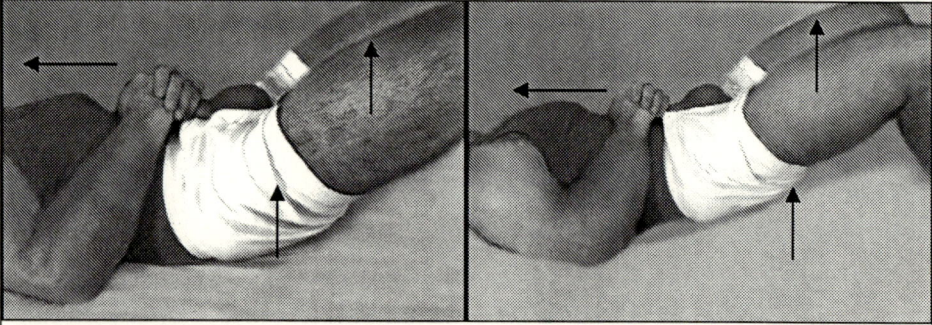

2- While uplifting your buttocks pull the penis toward your chest, then return to the first position.

33- Legs up Pull

Penis state: Flaccid
Target muscles: Lower Back, Abdominal, Arm
Penis strengths: Length increase
Safety: Do not put too much weight on your penis.
Repeat: 30 times

Lie down on your back.

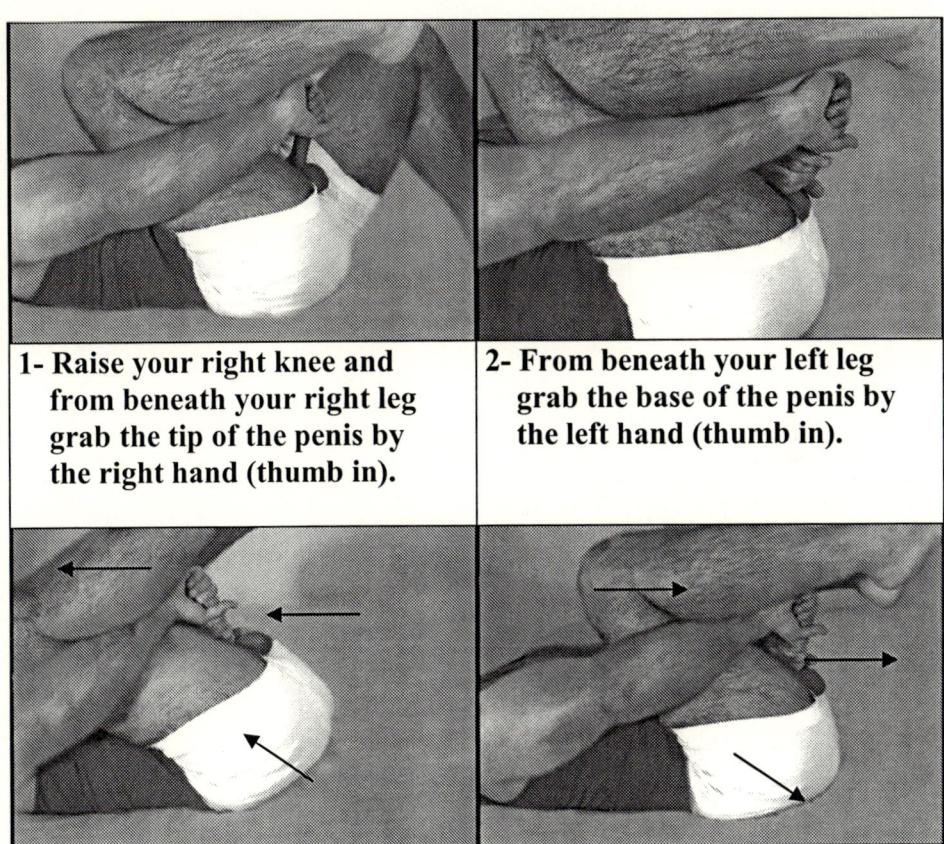

1- Raise your right knee and from beneath your right leg grab the tip of the penis by the right hand (thumb in).

2- From beneath your left leg grab the base of the penis by the left hand (thumb in).

3- Lift up your buttocks, and pull the penis and your legs simultaneously toward your chest, and then return to the first position.

Section 3

<u>Stand-up Lubricated Exercises</u>

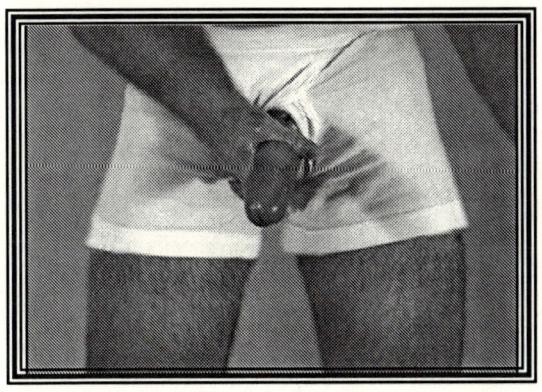

34- <u>Jelq Technique</u> (Milking)

Penis state: Lubricated, Semi erect
Target muscles: Arm, Chest
Penis strengths: Enlargement and increase in blood reservoir
Safety: Start with light pressure until the penis is warmed-up.
Remark: Jelqing is an ancient technique to enlarge penis.
Repeat: 50 times

Stand straight with legs slightly apart.

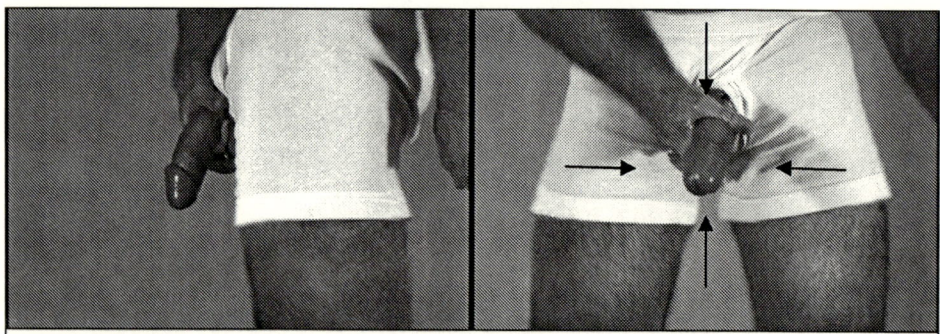

1- Grab the base of the penis by circling the thumb and the forefinger of your right hand around it (thumb out).

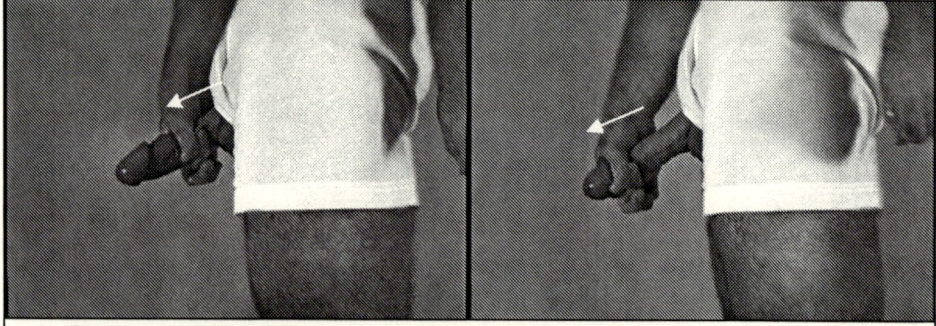

2- Slide your thumb and forefinger outward while squeezing the penis, and rushing the blood to the tip.

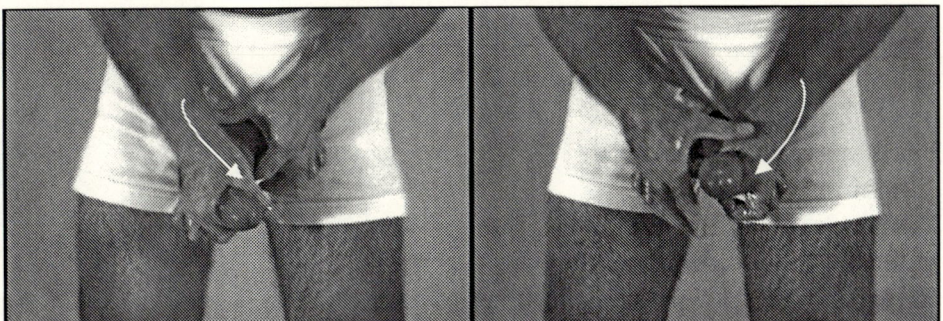

3- When your right hand reaches the tip of the penis add your left thumb and the index finger to the base to continually rush the blood to the tip.

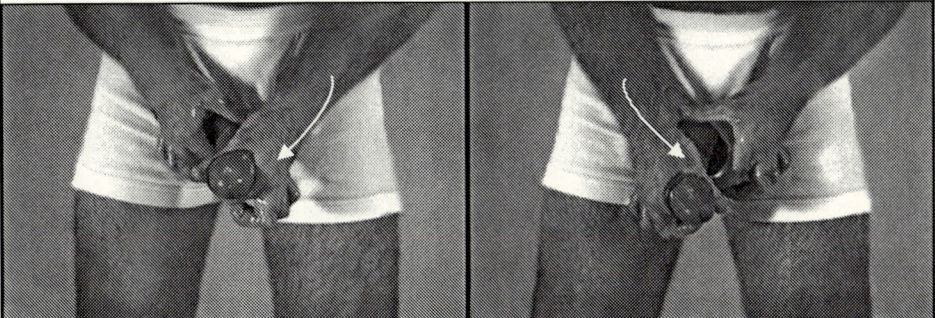

4- Alternate the two hands in a way that blood is constantly rushed to the tip of the penis.

35- Inflation Exercise

Penis state: Lubricated, Erect
Target muscles: Arm, Chest
Penis strengths: Base muscles, Thickness
Safety: Use enough lubrication to avoid friction.
Repeat: 25 times clockwise, 25 times counter clockwise

Stand straight with legs slightly apart.

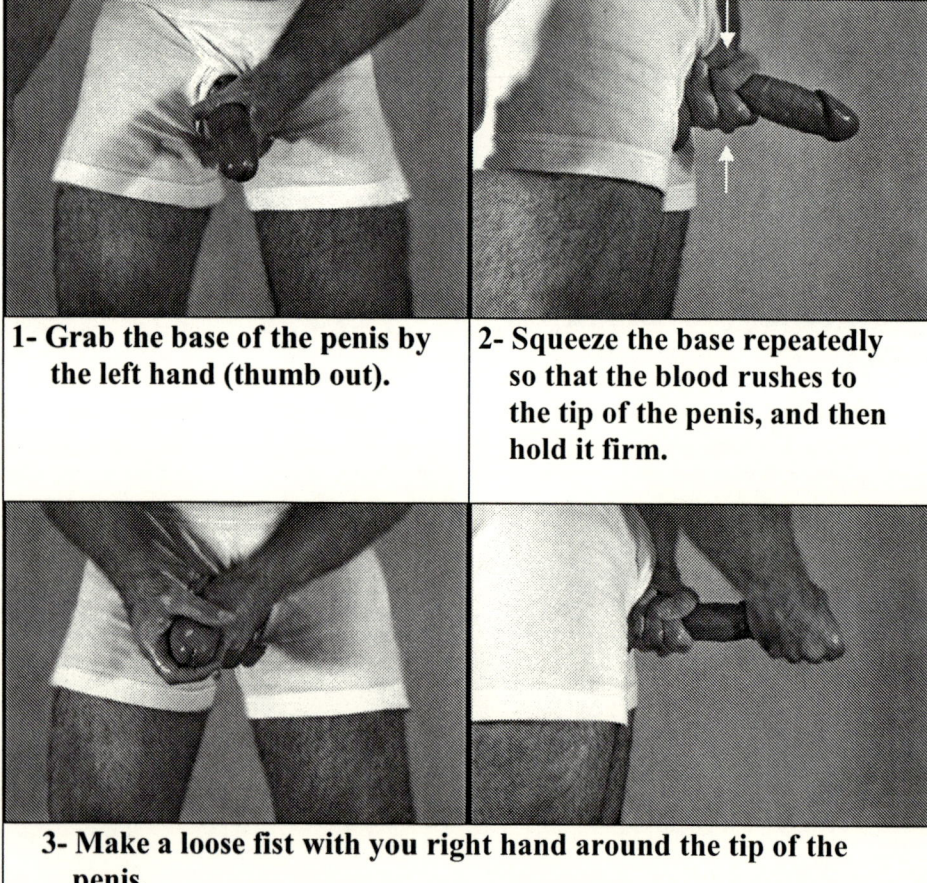

1- Grab the base of the penis by the left hand (thumb out).	2- Squeeze the base repeatedly so that the blood rushes to the tip of the penis, and then hold it firm.

3- Make a loose fist with you right hand around the tip of the penis.

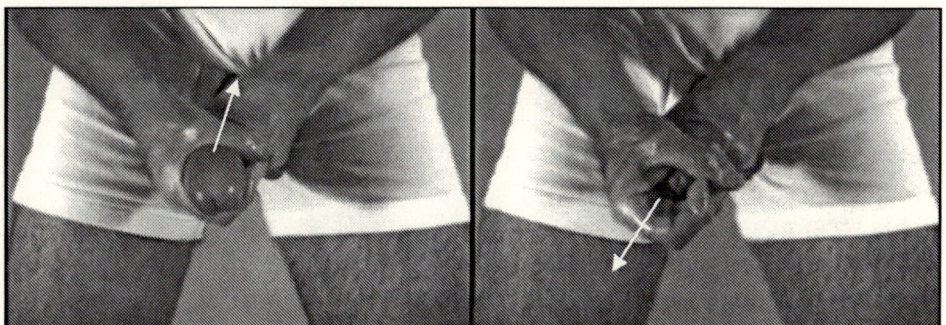

4- While the base of the penis is squeezed by your left hand, by your right hand and with the strength of your right arm and chest stroke in and out.

Repeat the whole exercise by switching hands.

36- Stroke Exercise

Penis state: Lubricated, Erect
Target muscles: Arm, Chest
Penis strengths: Thickness, General strength
Safety: Use enough lubrication to avoid friction.
Repeat: 25 times clockwise, 25 times counter clockwise

Stand straight with legs slightly apart.

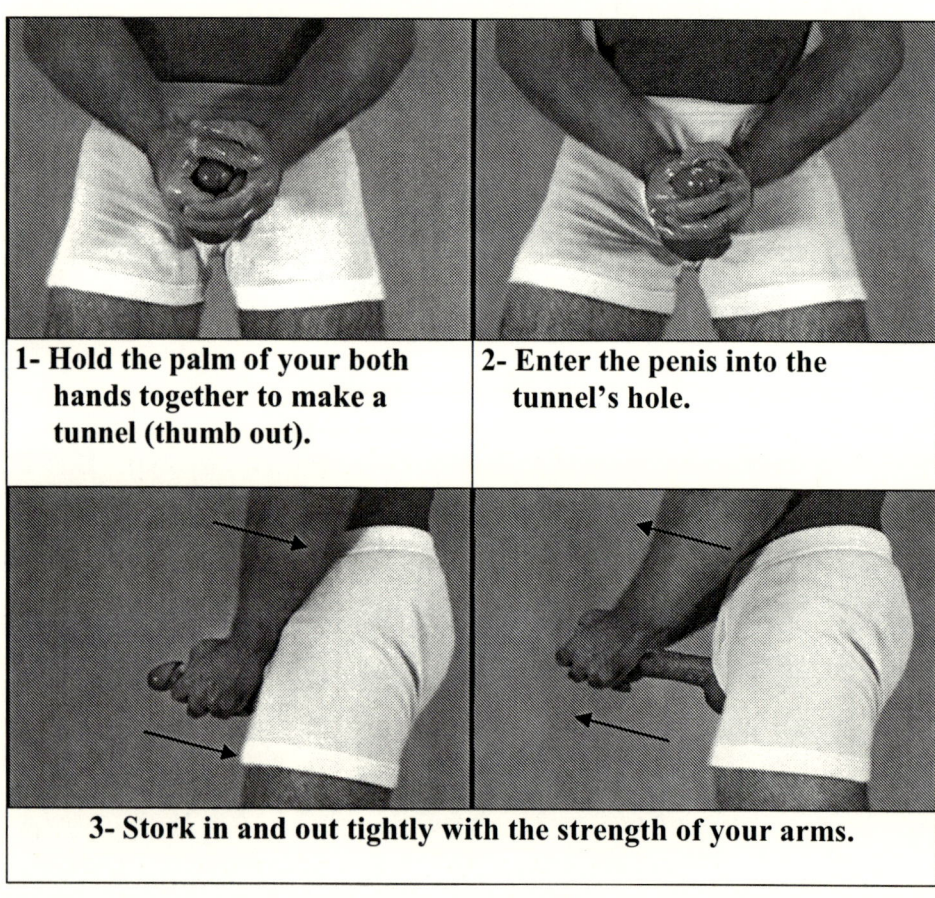

1- Hold the palm of your both hands together to make a tunnel (thumb out).

2- Enter the penis into the tunnel's hole.

3- Stork in and out tightly with the strength of your arms.

37- <u>Downward Milking</u>

Penis state: Lubricated, Semi erect
Target muscles: Arm, Chest
Penis strengths: Length increase, Thickness
Safety: Start with light pressure until the penis is warmed-up.
Repeat: 50 times

Stand straight with legs apart.

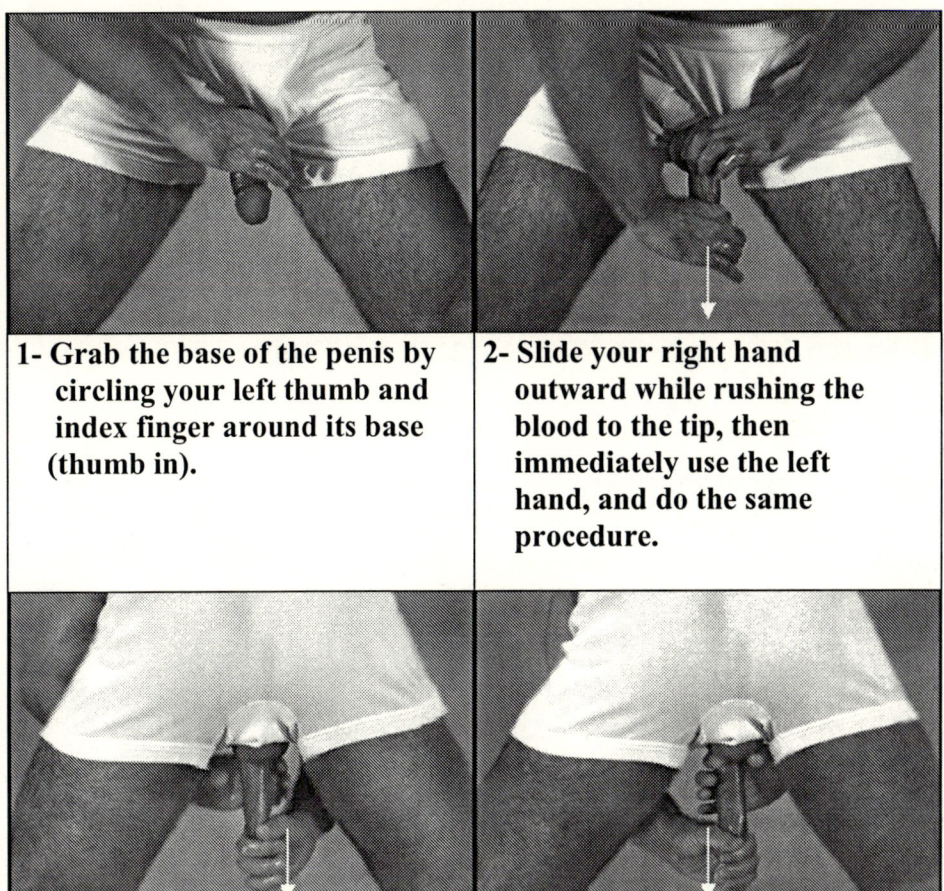

1- Grab the base of the penis by circling your left thumb and index finger around its base (thumb in).	2- Slide your right hand outward while rushing the blood to the tip, then immediately use the left hand, and do the same procedure.

3- Alternate the two hands to stretch the penis and to rush blood to the tip of the penis.

38- Under Leg Milking

Penis state: Lubricated, Semi erect
Target muscles: Arm, Chest
Penis strengths: Length increase, Thickness
Safety: Start with light pressure until the penis is warmed-up.
Repeat: 50 times

Raise your right knee and support your leg against a chair.

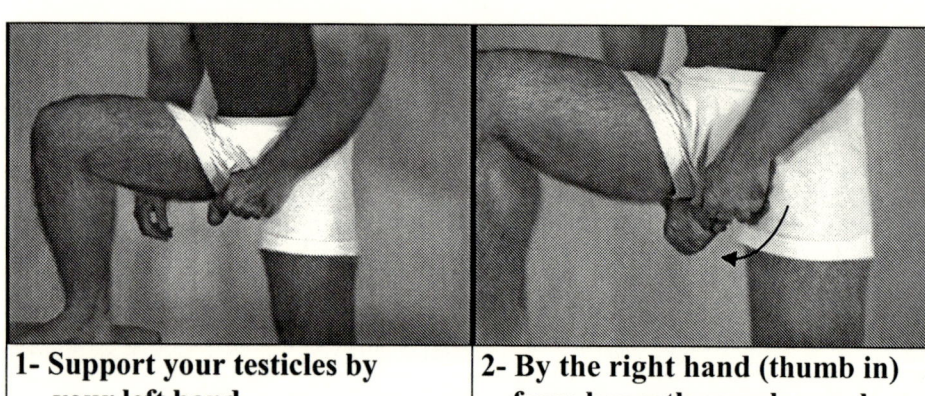

1- Support your testicles by your left hand.	2- By the right hand (thumb in) from beneath your leg grab the base of the penis.

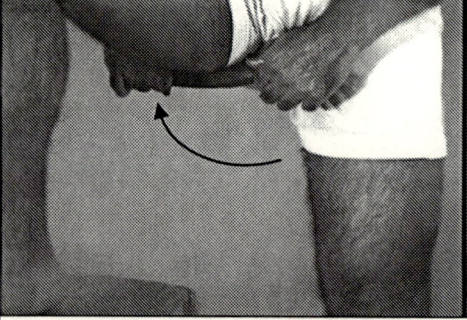 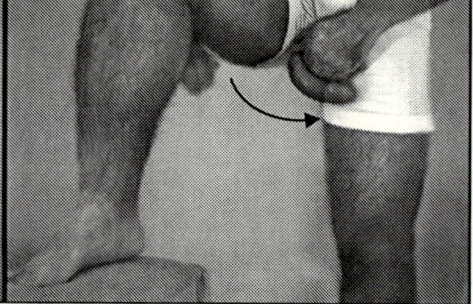

3- Then in an upward direction, beneath your leg, slide your fist toward the tip of the penis while rushing the blood to the tip, and then release the penis.

Repeat the whole exercise by your left hand and left leg.

84

39- **Behind Milking**

Penis state: Lubricated, Semi erect
Target muscles: Arm, Hand, Chest, Upper back
Penis strengths: Length increase, Thickness
Safety: Start with light pressure until the penis is warmed-up.
Repeat: 50 times

Raise your right knee and support your leg against a chair.

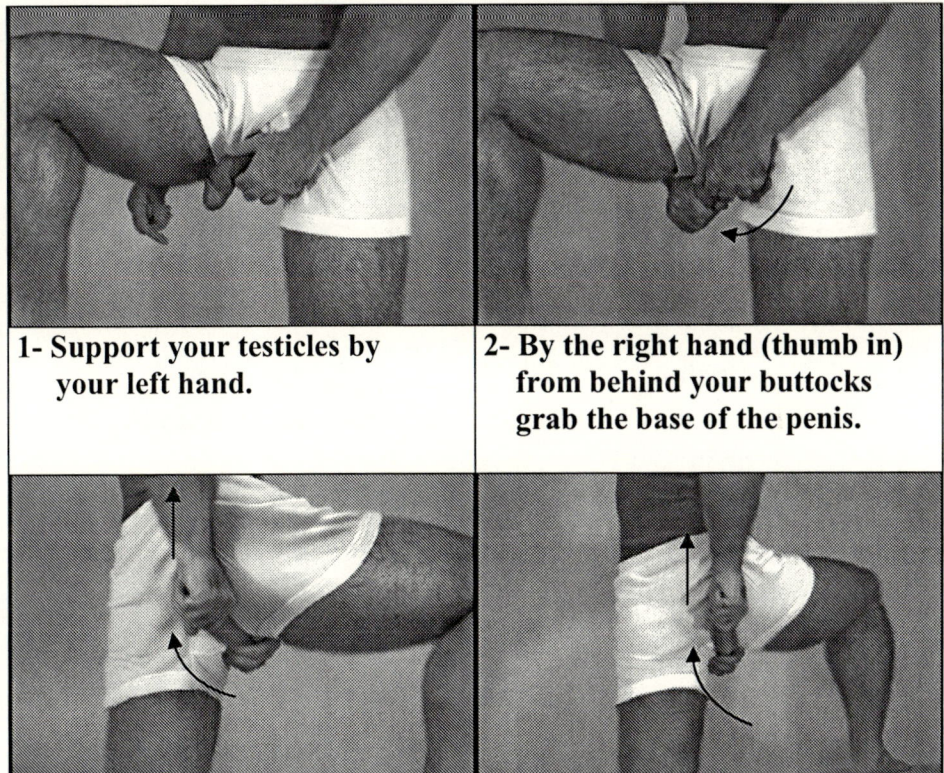

1- Support your testicles by your left hand.	2- By the right hand (thumb in) from behind your buttocks grab the base of the penis.

3- Then in an upward direction from behind slide your fist toward the tip of the penis while rushing the blood to the tip, and then release it.

Repeat the whole exercise by your left hand and left leg.

40- <u>Bend Milking</u>

Penis state: Lubricated, Erect
Target muscles: Arm, Hand, Chest
Penis strengths: Length increase, Thickness
Safety: Start with light pressure until the penis is warmed-up.
Repeat: 50 times

Stand straight with legs slightly apart.

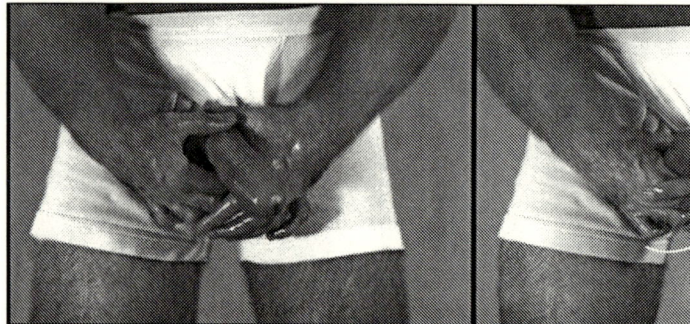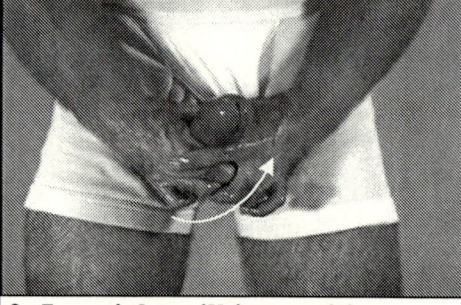

1- Make a tunnel by the attachment of both forefingers and index fingers (thumb out) and enter the penis fully into the hole.	2- In a tight milking position slide your hands toward the tip while bending the penis upward.

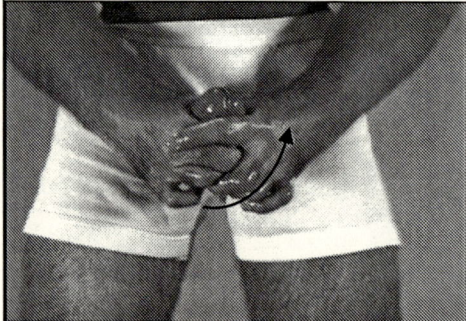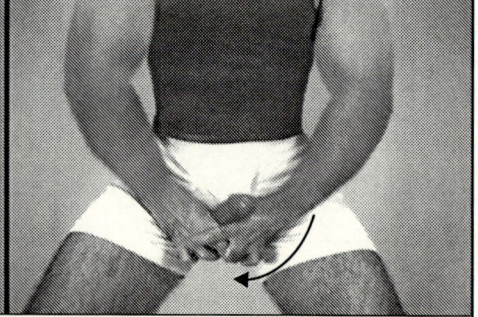

3- When your hand is at the tip of the penis return to the first position and repeat the same procedure.

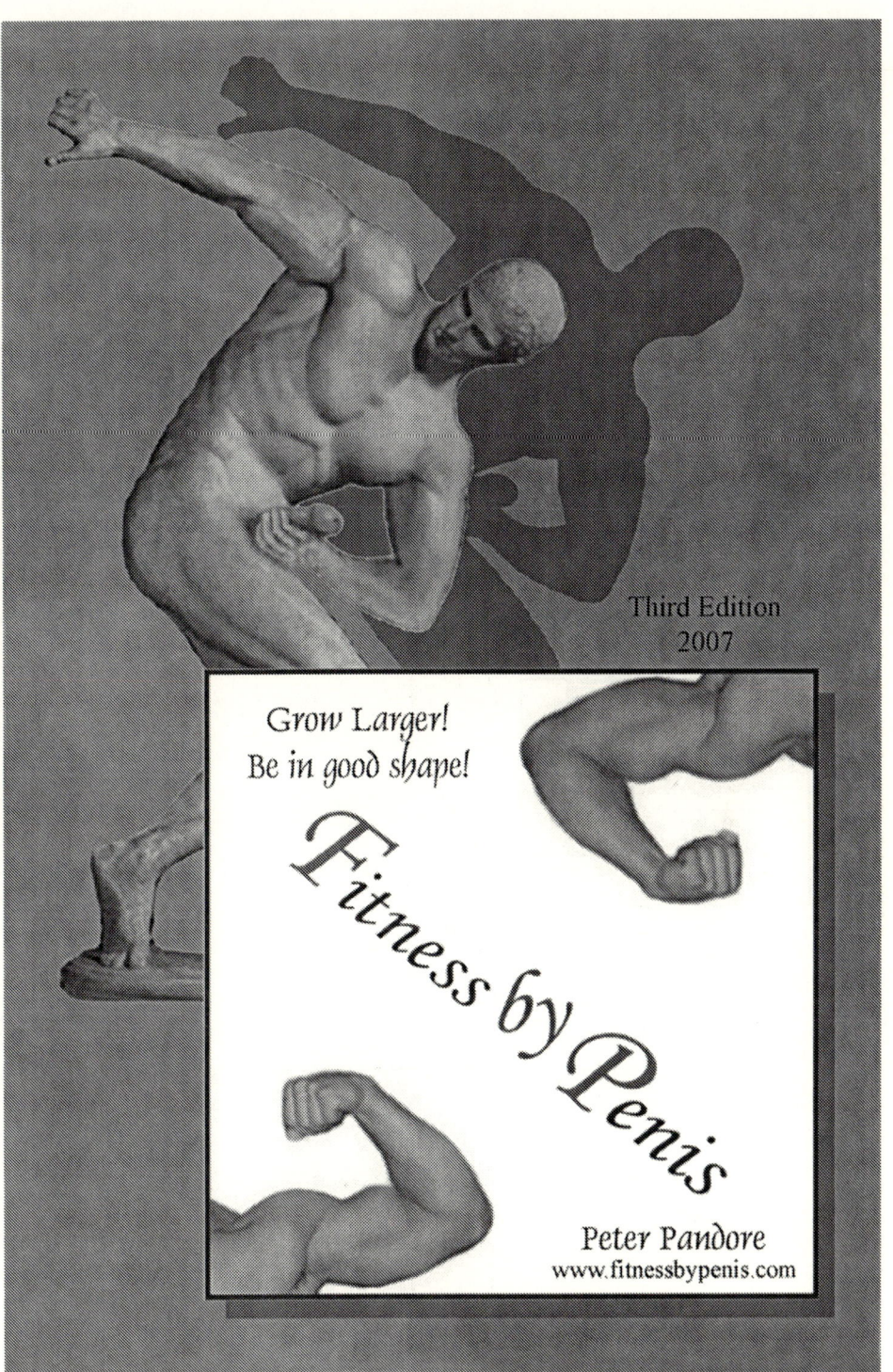

Third Edition
2007

Grow Larger!
Be in good shape!

Fitness by Penis

Peter Pandore
www.fitnessbypenis.com

Printed in the United Kingdom
by Lightning Source UK Ltd.
125726UK00002B/69/A

9 781411 699120